Survival
of the
Caregiver

A Treasury of ABC Self-Help Words
that Give Encouragement
and Support to the Caregiver

Janice Hucknall Snyder

Copyright 2015 by MSI Press, LLC

All rights reserved. No part of this book may be reproduced or utilized in any form or by any means, electronic or mechanical, including photocopying, recording, or by any information storage and retrieval system, without permission in writing from the publisher.

For information, contact

MSI Press
1760-F Airline Highway, #203
Hollister, CA 95023

Cover designed by Carl Leaver

Library of Congress Control Number: XXXXXXXX

ISBN: 978-1-942891-06-2

Dedication

I have heard of and known caregivers who died while devoting their lives to the care of a person with a catastrophic illness—an ironic and tragic ending. This book is dedicated to them and all those who have taken on the responsibility of caring for a loved one who is ill. This book is also dedicated to my husband, Richard, who fought the good fight. He took loving care of me for many years before it became my turn to care for him. My goal in writing this book is not only to help other caregivers like me survive, but to ease their burdens and actually improve their quality of life.

Janice Hucknall Snyder

Contents

Dedication iii

The Problem xi

Prologue xiii

A 15
Abilities – Acceptance – Accommodating – Achilles' Heel – Activities – Addictions – Adjustments – Advanced Directives – Advice – Agitation – Air Fresheners – Alcohol – Anger – Anxiety – Attitude

B 29
Backs – Back Rubs – Back-ups – Baking Soda – Bargains – Beautiful – Bedsores – Bed-Wetting – Belief – Blame – Blessings – Body Language – Boredom – Bowel Movements – Breaks – Budget

C 39
Calmness – Caring – Car Repairs – Changes – Choices – Church – Cleanliness – Comedy – Commitment – Common Sense – Communications – Compartments – Confronting – Copiers – Coping – C.P.R. – Credit – Crutches – Crying

D 51
Dancing – Day-Care Centers – Daydreams – Death – Debts – Decisions – Deed to the House – Dehydration – Deodorant – Depression – Diet – Discipline – Discomforts – Discouraged – Disruptions – Doubt – Dressing – Drooling – Duty

E 61
Efficiency – Emergencies – Empathy – Emotions – Encouragement – Energy – Ensure – Entertainment – Envy – Errors – Examinations – Exercise – Exhaustion – Experience

F 69
Facts of Life – Fairness – Family – Fear – Feelings – Fire – Flowers – Food – Forcefulness – Forgiveness – Freedom – Friends – Frustration – Fun – Future

G 81
Gentleness – Give and Take – Goals – Grief – Grip Bars – Grateful – Growing – Guilt

H 87
Habits – Hamstrings – Happiness – Health – Helplessness – Hobbies – Hope – Hospice – Holding and Hugging

I 93
Ice Cream – I.D. Bracelets – Illnesses – Impatience – Individuality – Insurance – Intercoms – Intercourse

J 101
Jargon – Jeopardy – Journal Keeping – Joyful Countenance – Judgment – Jumping Rope

K 105
Kaleidoscopes – Keys – Kindness – Kisses – Kitchens – Knowing – Knowledge

L 109
Labels – Laughter – Lawyers – Leisure – Limits – Listening – Little Things – Living Wills – Looking Ahead – Loving – Lows – Luck

M 117
Maintenance – Makeovers – Massages – Masturbation – Medicaid – Medicare Medications – Memories – Miracles – Moon – Murphy's Law – Music

N 127
Needs – Negative thinking – Neglect – Neighbors – Nervousness – Neutral – No –Noise – Nuisance – Nursing Home – Nutrition

O 135
Obligations – Obstacles – One Day at a time – Open-Mindedness – Ophthalmologists – Optimism – Organization – Outings – Overwhelmed

P 141
Patience of a Saint – Peace of Mind – People – Pets – Plan – Plastic – Positive Thinking – Power of Attorney – Prayer – Preparations – Prescriptions – Prevention – Priorities – Problems – Psychiatrists – Psychologists

Q 149
Quality of Life – Quantity Buying – Quarreling – Questions – Quiet time – Quitting

R..155
Reading – Reality – Receptiveness – Reconciling – Records – Regrets – Relationships – Relatives – Relaxing – Reminiscing – Repressing – Responsibilities – Rewards – Rushing

S 163
    Sacrificing – Schedules – Seclusion – Self-Control –
    Self-Esteem – Selfishness – Sharing – Shattered – Shoes
    – Shopping – Showers – Sing – Sleeping – Smile – Smoke
    Alarms – Solutions – Spirit – Stress – Success – Suicide –
    Supportive

T 177
    Tact – Teeth – Telephones – Television – Tempers – Time
    – Tiredness – Touching – Traveling – Trust – Try

U 183
    Unattended – Unawareness – Understanding – Unfairness
    – Unnatural and Unpleasant – Upsets – Urine

V 189
    Vacations – Variety – Videos, CDs and DVDs – Vegetables
    – Velcro – Vertigo – Viagra – Victory – Vigorous –
    Violence – Viruses – Vise-Like Grips – Vitamins – Voice

W 197
    Walking – Wandering – Weariness – Weather – Well-
    Being – Wheelchairs –Whining – Why? – Will-Power
    – Withdrawal – Wondering – Words – Working – World
    Happenings – Worrying – Worth – Writing

X 205
    X – X-Rays – X-Y-Z

Y..209
    Yearnings – Yelling – Yellow Brick Roads – Yesterday –
    Yoga – "You"

Z..213
    Zeal – Zenith – Zero – Zest – Zippers

In Closing 215

POSTSCRIPT 217

Select MSI Books 219

Janice Hucknall Snyder

Acknowledgements

I am deeply grateful to Betty Leaver, the Managing Editor, whose wisdom and encouragement was very meaningful.

I thank Mary Ann Raemisch, the Copy Editor, who did an excellent job, much appreciated.

For the artistic endeavors of Carl Leaver, in designing the thoughtful cover, I am sincerely pleased.

To my sister, Nanette Hucknall, author of "The Rose and the Sword", whose vast knowledge and support made this endeavor possible.

To my son-in-law, Randy Leonard, a computer expert and consultant, who formatted my book and gave great encouragement.

And last but not least, my granddaughter, Emily Leonard, who is a English A-Plus student and edited all the grammar in my book.

Janice Hucknall Snyder

The Problem

There are all kinds of debilitating illnesses that make it necessary for someone to take over the care of another person. It is usually a husband, wife, parent, son or daughter who is given this role in life.

Caring for another is an awesome responsibility, which is very complex and frightening. The person needing constant care could have become suddenly dependent, as in the case of strokes or auto and industrial accidents. Other illnesses, like Multiple Sclerosis, Cancer, Parkinson's disease, Rheumatoid Arthritis, Depression, Alzheimer's disease, or Dementia, can slowly progress over a period of many years. Still other people may have suffered a loss of vision or have experienced multiple aging problems. In any event, the caregiver has, whether suddenly or slowly, had his or her life altered profoundly. It is devastating from the aspect that the caregiver, in all probability, is a healthy, active, out-going and alert person who is required to be confined with someone who is ill, slowed-down or immobile, depressed and/or confused.

Janice Hucknall Snyder

Since the caregiver is first of all a human being, he or she has strengths and weaknesses too. Therefore, it is important to recognize and know one's own limits. Learning how to pace oneself is a key consideration when trying to survive the varied and constant duties involved in caring for someone with a catastrophic illness. Taking care of yourself physically, mentally and emotionally is a must.

Prologue

This is not a technical book. If your loved one has Alzheimer's Disease, Parkinson's Disease, Cystic Fibrosis, Heart Failure, Diabetes, Cerebral Palsy, or has experienced depression, a stroke, spinal injuries or any number of other debilitating catastrophic illnesses, there are many books in the library that describe all the problems, treatments, and prognoses of each of these conditions. Doctors and scholars who have specialized in these illnesses write these books. There is valuable information to be found in these accounts, and you should avail yourself to the ones pertaining to the particular problems of your loved one.

This is a book devoted to the caregivers of those with tragic illnesses. My twenty years of experience as a caregiver have given me many insights into coping with and surviving the problems that come with caring for an ill person. This book gives encouragement, along with valuable information I learned the hard way by trial and error. It is my hope that it will ease the way for caregivers going through this most difficult transition.

Janice Hucknall Snyder

I am a very private person. Some of the things I find essential to discuss in this book are difficult for me; they invade the privacy of my life and that of the loved one I am caring for. However, the importance of conveying, in open discussion, all the ramifications of surviving in the caregiver's world outweigh my privilege of privacy.

Each individual's circumstances are unique. Some of the things I have written about may not be relevant to your particular situation, but the book is very supportive in many different areas of a caregiver's life. My information comes from my experience of dealing, day by day, with another person, whom I deeply love and whom is totally dependent on me. A lot of my thoughts come from the heart openly, honestly and sincerely. I pray that the reader will find help, comfort and solace in my words and in the knowledge that others share the struggle, pain and even anger. We all deserve to survive the ordeal.

Doctors who write technical books sympathize with your circumstances and say they understand, but the only one who can really relate to what the caregiver's life is like, day in and day out, is another person walking in a pair of caregiver's shoes.

Come join me now for a walk through an alphabet of words, which will go a long way in helping you survive as a caregiver.

A

ABILITIES are unique and varied in each individual. I hope your parents let you become the person you were meant to be. Did they? If so, then you have developed your own interests. You have been given the opportunity of becoming a happy and well-adjusted person. In which case, you are now better prepared mentally to deal with your current role as caregiver. In fact, all the problems that face you during your lifetime will be more manageable.

It is a tragedy when a child is expected to follow in his/her parent's footsteps. Many times, it leads to failure, depression and even self-destruction. Ultimately, some of these people end up requiring a caregiver—sad but true.

When you are comfortable with who you are, you are better able to respond in affirmative ways to all others. When your life is smothered in negative thoughts and feelings, you are trapped within yourself. That makes it very difficult to be giving and cheerful when caring for someone who is confined.

As a caregiver, it is important to keep your mind open to receiving and accepting happiness, no matter what the circumstances. You need to continue to use your God-given abilities to grow and enjoy who you are.

ACCEPTANCE of what is unalterable is half the battle. When my husband became disabled with Parkinson's disease and then developed the complications of Dementia, it was truly difficult to accept the circumstances in which I found myself. I finally came to realize that constantly fretting about what had happened to our lives wouldn't change one thing. What you can't change from without, you have to change from within. I could not change what had happened to my husband, but I could change how I perceived it. Acceptance helped me deal with the circumstances in a positive way. Positive thinking is very important when giving hope and encouragement to the disabled and to yourself.

ACCOMMODATING means adapting. This is something caregivers need to keep in mind. The more you simplify daily procedures, the more time is left over for personal activities. If there are time-consuming problems within your daily routine, stop and think about how they could be done with less difficulty. Often, the solution is so simple that it is overlooked. Ask other people how they would handle the problem. Someone who is less involved, day in and day out, may see the answer immediately.

I had a big problem keeping the fitted sheet on my husband's bed from pulling loose every night. The sheet and the plastic protective cover underneath the sheet would slip off easily because of my husband's tossing and turning. One day, a mail-order catalog arrived at the house (order one item and you are on everyone's list forever). Catalogs are fun to look through and can give you good ideas. This particular magazine pictured elastic garters to put on the corners of the sheets to keep them in place. I ordered some, thinking my problem was solved. Wrong. They worked fine, but since I had to change the sheets frequently, I found putting the garters on and off laborious.

Another catalog arrived later. Another possibility. This time I ordered Styrofoam fitted corners. I put the garters on the plastic mattress cover to hold it firmly. Then, the Styrofoam corners went on each corner of the fitted bottom sheet. The Styrofoam corners took a second to put on and take off, but they worked great. Problem solved? Well, yes, but sometime later I realized I could just sew bands of elastic to the corners of the sheets permanently. That was better yet. Still later, someone told me if I just added an extra pad to the protective covering at nighttime, it would keep the sheet from even getting wet and needing to be changed at all. So, through trial, error, and adaptation, solutions were found. The solutions saved me time, energy, and loads of frustration.

Be accommodating to yourself. Think about the daily chores that are the biggest hassles. Try a different way—adapt.

ACHILLES' HEEL Do you have one? Most of us do. However, we don't always want to recognize our own vulnerability. Are you too quick to anger, do you become overemotional, are you easily offended, are you a procrastinator, or perhaps, are you all of these? If you weren't before you were a caregiver, you probably are now.

Maybe your "weak spot" is not being able to say "no" to anyone. If so, you are in big trouble. With your hectic schedule, there should be no qualms about saying, "Sorry, no can do," to family and friends. People who love and care about you will not have their feelings hurt. The rest don't count. If you don't learn to say "no," you will probably wear out long before the person you are caring for does.

Janice Hucknall Snyder

ACTIVITIES that allow caregivers to grow in their personal lives are a real lifesaver. Reading is at the top of the list for many reasons. It takes you on a wonderful adventure, leaving cares far behind. Reading costs nothing, exercises your grey matter, and can be done at home.

Reading aloud to the confined person is an enjoyable pastime for two. Audio books from the library are a wonderful way to occupy your loved one while you are busy with other duties.

Hopefully, you had some hobbies before this confinement occurred. Make a point of not neglecting or sacrificing these activities, especially now. Schedule hobby time even if it's only half an hour a day.

I've played bridge with three people for 32 years. We took turns going to each other's homes once a week. A minor adjustment made it possible for me to continue playing; my girlfriends agreed to come to my house every Wednesday night for our bridge party. They didn't mind waiting when it was time for me to put Richard to bed. In fact, they would talk so fast and furious that we were hardly missed.

Keep your interests alive. Activities are still possible when you are flexible.

ADDICTIONS are not limited to drugs, alcohol, and food although these are three of the most devastating and prevalent. People are addicted to lots of other things, even lying. I always thought it would be great if habitual liars really did grow long noses just like Pinocchio. Then, we could spot them and stay clear. Plastic surgeons sure would have a thriving business, wouldn't they?

Many people are addicted to work. They never stop to smell the roses, feel the sea spray on their face as they walk along the shore, read bedtime stories to their children, or do any number of other beautiful things that are more important than working a 16-hour hour day.

As a caregiver, you can become a workaholic with your heavy schedule requirements. You need to separate and regulate the "must dos" from the "should dos," such as: a wet bed must be changed and the furniture should be dusted. (I never did like dusting, and now I have a good excuse.)

A person with a lot of excess nervous energy (that's me) tends to do it all. This frustrates family and friends who would like to help out, too, if given the chance. I guess that makes me an "I can do it myself" addict, which is contradictory to surviving as a caregiver. I am improving, though. Recently, my daughter, the nurse, said that since she had four days off, she wanted to spend one of them with her dad and have dinner ready for me when I got home from work. I actually said, "That would be great."

Normally, I would have said, "Oh no, you're pregnant, and once the baby arrives you will have little time for yourself," but things aren't normal when you're a caregiver. It means a lot to get a break. I gladly accepted her thoughtful offer. More important, I realized that our daughter needed and cherished the opportunity to have time alone with her dad.

The consideration here is to moderate your undertakings, then you won't become addicted and you won't become blind to what is important for you and those you love.

ADJUSTMENTS in living conditions for a disabled person are ongoing. Keeping a close eye on your patient helps you determine when adjustments might be necessary and can prevent accidents.

Janice Hucknall Snyder

I had to do a lot of adjusting recently. It was something I had put off for a long while because I was dreading it. My husband was getting harder and harder to get up the stairs at night. A frightening experience convinced me to adjust in a hurry. I had gotten him halfway up the stairs when he froze and then started pushing backwards. All I could do was hold him to keep us both from falling. After ten minutes, which seemed more like an hour, I talked him into relaxing and going on up. The next day, a bed was moved downstairs to my study, now renamed "Richard's Bedroom." Closets and cabinets were cleared of various, sundry junk and replaced with his clothes and other essentials. The grip bars from upstairs were attached in strategic places downstairs. A new showerhead with a hose was installed in the downstairs shower, and I became an all-night "couch potato," sleeping in the living room. My study is now in the kitchen—always my favorite room, anyway. To my surprise, being on one floor has made life much easier. Now I'm glad I adapted.

Changes are difficult at best, but when you realize that someone's safety is at risk, sooner is better.

ADVANCED DIRECTIVES give you and your dependent control over the extent of treatments implemented on your bodies while in a hospital. These directives are required by many hospitals upon admission. The forms can be obtained from the hospital and filled out prior to being admitted for some conditions. Basically, the patient or guardian states the patient's wishes concerning the extent of treatments given, directing at which point the individual wishes treatment to be discontinued. The advanced directive is only activated in terminally ill patients. It is not necessary to have the paper notarized, just witnessed.

Hospital rules vary in different parts of the country. Check in your area for the correct procedure. It is easier for all concerned to fill out this form before there is any real need. Keep a copy in your safe deposit box, as well as in the house and with another family member.

The only real difference between an advanced directive and a living will (see under "L") is that the advanced directive is required by the hospital upon admission for an illness or surgery while the living will is something you can have written up when you are in good health so that, in the event of a sudden illness, like a stroke or automobile accident, your wishes will be carried out even though you are not able to verbalize them.

ADVICE can be constructive or destructive, needed or not needed, wanted or not wanted, taken or not taken. Since this book contains a lot of advice, I'm hoping that it is constructive, needed, wanted, and taken. Learn to recognize the difference.

I would have trouble taking advice on caregiving from a person who has never had to care for a parent, partner, or child. How could he or she possibly relate to the emotional trauma, pain and physical management problems a caregiver encounters? However, most people have had some experience in caring, so it is wise to keep an open mind when others offer advice. Every bit helps if it's constructive, and the only way to find that out is to listen.

AGITATION in the dependent should be dealt with immediately and calmly, but firmly. Alzheimer's patients get very frustrated, and their agitation is certainly understandable. When they are in this state, they can become very angry and very strong. Be aware that outbursts can come on suddenly, without warning. And don't for one moment think that your kind and gentle mate would never do such a thing as strike or kick you. This is not the same loving person you've shared a lifetime with. He doesn't know he's supposed to love you. He doesn't even know who you are at this point. He is enraged and striking out to vent that anger. So, be alert to the possibility of such an outburst. The first time it happens is shocking and very unsettling.

You have a responsibility to get help if the situation warrants it. There are medications that will calm the patient, and they should be utilized. In cases where your well-being is at risk and medications are not controlling the problem, it is necessary to find a facility to take over the care of your loved one. This is a sad reality. There is a time for giving and a time for giving over. Look into other arrangements as soon as outbursts begin to become more aggressive. Be cautious, and be prepared.

AIR FRESHENERS take up a whole shelf in the grocery store. They come in all shapes and sizes, solids and sprays. The circumstances of one particular day were such that none of the sprays I used were effective. The odor persisted. Then, my thoughtful cousin, Caroline, brought me a gift that was more appreciated than a dozen roses would have been. It was a freshener that plugs into the wall socket. When it heats up, the "pleasant" scent wins out. It permeates the room completely and adequately for three months. I had never heard about this product, but how happy I was that she had! Air fresheners are an important addition to your home, especially if you want visitors to come more than once.

A word of caution, I've been informed that most air fresheners contain chemicals. Many patients may have adverse reactions to these chemicals. If you suspect these chemicals might cause changes in your patient's condition, discontinue use of air fresheners. Instead, use good ol' baking soda, or quarter an onion and put the pieces in four bowls of water placed in needed areas. It works.

ALCOHOL can and does destroy people. I don't think I've ever turned down a margarita in my whole life, well maybe if I've already had two. Fortunately, my husband and I have never had a problem with alcohol. We have enjoyed an occasional cocktail before dinner, offered drinks to friends dropping by and imbibed at parties. I still do all of the above, but unfortunately, my husband cannot. Now his medications and condition require total abstinence. When he was still able to attend parties, I made sure the host knew ahead of time to fix a non-alcoholic beverage. That way he felt included in the festivities, and there were no repercussions. Our friends understood the situation and knew the recipe for my husband's drink.

If you know you have a drinking problem and cannot control your thirst for alcohol, you should seek help immediately. Run, do not walk, to your nearest Alcoholics Anonymous meeting. A caregiver's responsibilities require total alertness at all times. A tendency to overindulge "socially" can grow into a serious problem. Caregivers under constant stress are vulnerable. Don't put yourself or your loved one in jeopardy.

ANGER needs to be verbalized and needs an outlet. Show me a caregiver who says he or she never gets angry, and I'll show you a liar or a saint.

Once, a patient who was 75 years old came into my office. She had been caring for her 97-year-old mother for ten years. I told her I was a caregiver, too, and remarked that I thought caring for someone else when you were 75 must be most difficult. With a sheepish look on her face she said, "You know, I'm ashamed to tell you this, but sometimes I get very angry."

I responded, "Of course you do; that's only natural. I get angry, too." She looked astonished.

"You do?" she said, "I thought I was the only one." I couldn't believe my ears. I assured her that most caregivers experience this strong emotion more often than they would like to admit. She was very happy and relieved to hear that.

There is no way you can keep from feeling angry about seeing your loved one suffering and about having acquired such tremendous responsibilities, all while losing your precious freedom.

It is okay to feel angry, but don't harbor your anger; it isn't safe. Don't let anger turn you into a resentful person for that will hurt you both. Do find a close friend, a buddy you can trust to keep what you say confidential, and unload your tales of woe on this understanding, patient soul, and be thankful for him or her. If no such individual is within easy grasp, consider joining one of the many support groups that are available in most communities. The local newspaper usually runs a long list of these, giving the times and dates of the meetings where everyone is welcome. Hearing other people sharing their feelings of anger and frustration will make you realize you are not alone. That's a good feeling. You find out you have not become some terrible monster for having these feelings. On the contrary, you are still the same good person. You are simply dealing with great adversity. If your circumstances are such that getting out of the house to attend meetings is a near impossibility, then take another action. Jump into a hot shower and scream and cry until you feel in control again, or do a workout of floor exercises, but get that anger out before it does you in.

ANXIETY is unavoidable when dealing with a catastrophic illness. The big question is how to keep your anxiety to a minimum so that the disabled person doesn't pick up on it and get anxious, too. You cannot avoid having times of great anxiety when your loved one's illness develops complications. It can become so devastating.

Then, there's the matter of money, the lack of which causes plenty of anxiety. Money doesn't grow on trees, but if it did, caregivers certainly would be up there plucking it off. The drugs alone can be a terrible financial burden. My husband's medications cost over $600 a month and are only partially covered by my supplemental insurance. You can apply for Social Security disability benefits before age 65, and this does help a lot with these kinds of expenses. If you have not already done so, you should make an appointment at once to get all the paperwork done. The Social Security office always has a large backlog of applicants, and each case must be researched and verified. It could be many months before your paperwork even reaches the top of the pile so that it can be considered.

Anxiety can give you ulcers, high blood pressure, or both if you don't already have them. Keep occupied with good books or a hobby so you don't dwell on your problems continuously. Remember, yesterday's cares are over and done, and tomorrow's cares are yet to come. Just do the best you can with today; that is all you really have and all you can really handle. Relax; take slow, deep breaths when the pressures close in on you.

There are medications that the disabled person can be given to keep anxiety at a manageable level. Anxiety attacks are enervating and depressing to a person with a debilitating illness. They are a very real and difficult condition for you to deal with. Seek help from a doctor to ease this burden on yourself.

Janice Hucknall Snyder

ATTITUDE need improving? How you react to what is happening to you depends a lot on your attitude. When one woman was asked if the glass is half full or half empty, she replied, "I think it is just one more thing I'll have to wash."

Have you always been negative or positive, pessimistic or optimistic? If prior to the illness of the dependent person, you were an optimist, you will find it easier to survive. If you were a pessimist, your work is cut out for you. Keeping a positive frame of mind is extremely difficult when you are a negative thinker.

A good attitude is important in every area of your life. A happy spirit makes it possible to stay cheerful when caring for someone. This will, in turn, help to keep up the spirits of the disabled person. No, it's not always easy to do—how well I know—but when I'm down, the extra effort to be up usually results in everything going better.

Because you are an individual, you will have your own way of dealing with problems, including illness. I have worked in a doctor's office for years. I never cease to be amazed at the different ways people handle their illnesses. Some patients will be negative, helpless and demanding, while others are upbeat, smiling and courageous.

I remember one 60-year-old lady who had amputations of both legs well above the knees. When I attempted to help lift her from her wheelchair to the examining chair, she stopped me and said, "Thank you, but I don't need any help. I can do just fine all by myself." With that, she swung her torso up and around, kerplop! She landed right in the middle of that table. I was literally left standing with my mouth hanging open in amazement.

Oddly enough, I have noticed that the severity of a patient's problem is not a determining factor in that person's attitude. Some of the most handicapped patients have the sweetest dispositions. Others, far less impaired, can be downright surly.

There are differences in caregiver's attitudes, too. The temperamental patient may have a kind, loving caregiver, a true saint on earth. On the other hand, the gentle patient may have an angry, resentful caregiver. Granted, some of the patients are on their best behavior for the public. Meanwhile, at home they are giving their caregivers good cause to blow their top. Likewise, some of the 'saintly' caregivers in public are not always so kind on the home front. Our human imperfection is showing.

Which brings me to the point I want to make about having a good attitude to survive being a caregiver. Obviously, you can't always be Mr. or Ms. Sunshine. That would not be possible or even normal. But you do need to keep working at doing things that give your spirit a boost. When your spirits are up, so is your attitude. Things happen during the course of caring to knock the pins out from under you. Declare war on them! Fight back! Arm yourself with as much happiness as you can gather at any given time. Store up happy memories, and then draw on them when you are reaching the end of your rope. They will help to pull you through the tough times.

Janice Hucknall Snyder

B

BACKS are the mainstay of our bodies when they're in. When they go out on us, we are in big trouble as caregivers. The first time I pulled a muscle in my back, I was miserable for a week. Then, I forgot all about it and lifted something incorrectly again. Two weeks of misery followed. There are rules to live by when lifting something or someone: Always bend the knees and use the leg muscles, not the back. For better leverage, get as close to the object or person as possible. Leaning into the patient's torso minimizes back strain when helping to lift the patient to a sitting position or out of the bed. A slant board enables you to slide a person from and to a bed or chair with less lifting involved. If the dependent is a heavy person, try getting a medical lift that does most of the work.

There are special fabric braces made now that provide excellent support for your back. They wrap around the waist and are easily attached with Velcro. If you have to do a lot of moving and lifting of your dependent, it would be well worth it to invest in this kind of back support. Do exercises to strengthen your back muscles. Be sensible; avoid unnecessary lifting. Your back will thank you by keeping you straight and pain-free.

BACK RUBS are crucial and essential for the dependent if bed-ridden. They help to improve circulation and prevent bedsores. It is easier to rub backs than to take care of bedsores.

Similarly, caregivers constantly use their backs when caring for the patient and doing chores. If someone gives you a nice back rub, it's a real treat. I hope you know that kind of someone. The next best thing for those aches and pains is a long soak in the tub.

BACK-UPS are people you can call in a pinch or emergency. Family and friends living nearby should be familiar with your routine. They need to know the dosages and times for dispensing medications. Keep the schedule posted in a convenient place. Knowing others who can take over quickly with minimal instruction will reduce stress should you have to leave suddenly.

BAKING SODA gets a ten for versatility. It is good for making Toll House cookies, cleaning your teeth, calming acid indigestion, deodorizing the refrigerator and rooms, and sprinkling on urine spots in the rug. Accidents do happen. I keep a big box of baking soda handy in the bedroom. Not only does it deodorize the rug, it minimizes the staining, too.

BARGAINS we all love to find. They help to keep your wallet from having that empty look. Shop around for such items as Depends, talcum powder, moist towelettes, plastic bag liners and detergents for washing bed linens. Always buy in large quantities. Check the newspaper for specials. Cut out and use those pain-in-the-neck coupons—every bit helps. The large wholesale clubs usually have the best buys.

BEAUTIFUL is what life is supposed to be. The caregiver sees and lives with a part of life that, let's face it, isn't beautiful. The reality of a catastrophic illness is dependency on another, mental and physical suffering, and an altered, struggling lifestyle. What is beautiful is the shared love, courage, support, and understanding that two individuals can give to one another. That is what eases the burden for the caregiver and the dependent.

BEDSORES can become a serious problem for someone totally confined to their bed. I have not had to deal with this problem yet, so I consulted the doctor I work for.

A bed-ridden person should be rolled every 2-3 hours to prevent bedsores. A special egg-crate mattress helps to keep the air circulating underneath the patient. If patchy redness is seen, a doughnut-shaped cushion can be placed under the area to relieve the pressure. If blisters form, a physician should be consulted. These kinds of problems involve additional medical treatment, time and expense. Knowledge gained before a problem arises for the disabled person is always of benefit to the caregiver as well as the patient.

BED-WETTING keeps the washer going. The problem is not always solved entirely by using Depends or similar protections although they do help. If you are willing and able to get up 1-2 times a night to assist the disabled with bathroom needs, then a diaper is usually adequate. I find having my sleep interrupted during the night makes rising and shining at 5:15 a.m. very difficult. I prefer to strip the sheets in the morning, but to each his own in this department. It helps to have a system for handling this unpleasant task. I keep everything lined up within easy reach. I can almost do the changing in my sleep; in fact, I think I have at times.

Six months after writing this section on bed-wetting, someone suggested using double diapers or an extra padded insert at night, which is a simple solution. Why didn't I think of that? Works like a charm. It reduced the bed changing 90%. That smart advice was a tremendous time and energy saver and really appreciated.

Sometimes, the disabled person becomes confused during the night and tries to take the diaper off. Now, there's a scenario I'm familiar with. It looks like there's been a snowstorm inside the bedroom. Bits of wet cotton are everywhere, so I don a pair of my trusty rubber gloves and gather up the "snow."

Try to limit the amount of liquids ingested by the patient after 6 p.m. Remember: decreased intake, means decreased output!

BELIEF in a higher power gives strength and support to the caregiver. It is desperately needed at times. Each individual's spiritual life and inner faith is a very personal thing. However, when there is no one else near to turn to, there is great comfort in knowing you can turn to God. He is always just a prayer away.

There is also someone else it helps to believe in: yourself. Confidence and growing security with who you are as an individual come through your experience of life's challenges. Being a caregiver isn't just a burdensome duty. Through caring for another, you can find a special meaning for your own life.

BLAME can be a heavy load to bear. When things go wrong in life, don't get bogged down in blaming yourself or blaming someone else saying, "If only I had. . ." or, "If only you had. . ." Either way, blame can be destructive.

When something happens to a loved one, there is a tendency for others to take the blame. This is especially so when suicide is involved. Another person's choice is a heavy burden for you to bear. Think about that. Free yourself from senseless guilt because it will destroy you.

BLESSINGS are easy for me to expound on. How about you? My husband and I have had many blessings through the years: four wonderful children (a couple of miracles included) and loyal family members and friends; God bless each and every one. Whenever I'm feeling sorry for myself, I start counting my blessings. Before long, I've lost count and forgotten what I was feeling so down about. No matter who you are, things could always be worse and may even be worse one day. Remember, bad times do not last forever. Keep the faith. Believe what you are doing is the very best that you can do for right now because it truly is. Be thankful for all the opportunities and all the blessings in your life. Have you counted them lately?

BODY LANGUAGE communicates people's inner feelings and emotional attitudes toward one another. The way you stand, sit, make eye contact and gesture with your hands can convey a lot without one word spoken. You may not even be aware that your body is telling on you because these are unconscious gestures.

When you are feeling down, your mouth turns down, and the hugs and handholding are missed. Your patient will sense something is wrong and think he is the cause, which is probably right. That will put both of you in a slump. Negative body language will do that.

A good, upbeat attitude is also reflected in your body language. Your loved one will instinctively know and feel more relaxed and comfortable as a result. This, in turn, will reduce stress in your dependent, which always makes caregiving easier for you, the caregiver.

BOREDOM can set in when your life is confined to a routine of continuously caring for another. If your patient has had a stroke or has Alzheimer's disease, conversation tends to be very limited, but there should be more than, "Honey, take your pills," or, "Time for your pills, sweetheart," or "Pill time." Discuss different things even if it is all one-sided and sounds like a soliloquy. Your patient may be able to understand a lot more than you think.

When communications are limited, it is up to you to keep from being bored. Watch television and read. Stay in touch with people. Invite a neighbor in for afternoon tea, and chat on the phone with friends daily. Contact with people keeps the outside world open for you.

While we are on the subject of boredom, remember not to be boring yourself. When visiting with people, don't spend all the time boo-hooing about your lot in life or talking about the dependent's problems. That defeats the whole purpose. Discuss new and interesting subjects; get outside yourself.

If the other party asks about the person in your care, a brief discussion is appropriate. Graphic details are hard to digest and can turn people off. If your friends start disappearing into the woodwork, you know you overdid it.

BOWEL MOVEMENTS are a necessary bodily function, I'm afraid.

I had an uncle in his eighties, and when his daughter was out of town, I would make daily phone calls to check up on him. It never failed that before the conversation was concluded, he would tell me what a wonderful bowel movement he had had that day. I always congratulated him because it seemed expected, but I never really understood his need to discuss such a personal thing or his elation over it, until now. When someone is disabled, their whole system slows down, and normal, regular bowel habits slow down, too.

Someone else's bowels had never really interested me. I was shocked the first time I realized I had to make them a concern. Then, I was worried. It had been several days since I could remember anything happening in that department. So, I went to the drug store and bought some capsules that were supposed to do the trick. Nothing happened. Now, I was really worried. I had heard about people becoming impacted and going to the hospital to be freed up. Next, the druggist said to use a suppository. There was no immediate action, so I repeated the procedure. At last, the required results occurred, much to our mutual relief.

The doctor I work with suggested that I use rubber gloves for "special occasions" when laxatives have to be given. He donated a box to the cause—truly a gift of the greatest magnitude. Do keep disposable, rubber gloves handy; they make unpleasant clean-ups a whole lot more bearable. The gloves can be purchased at any medical supply company. Discount stores, such as K-Mart and Wal-Mart, often carry rubber gloves in the pharmaceutical or beauty sections at a lower price, so check around.

When constipation is a problem, talk to your doctor or trusty druggist. Stool softeners help, and if worse comes to worst, a Fleet's enema will usually get the job done.

A patient told me her mother became impacted. She had to don rubber gloves and manually extract some of the stool. Then she gave her a Fleet's enema, followed by more extracting. That is not a pleasant task for the caregiver and even less so for the disabled person. The point I want to make is that keeping track of bodily functions is a very critical part of caring for the disabled. Don't let too much time go by before taking some kind of action. What goes in must come out, or else you've got trouble.

BREAKS you want, if they are the lucky kind. You can't get enough of those. But breaks, as in fractures, are an unfortunate occurrence you would rather not have to deal with at all.

My husband often becomes disoriented. There are times when he doesn't watch where he's going, or he starts to sit down on air, thinking he's at his chair. Other times, he freezes when walking. He has tripped over things and broken ribs in a couple of bad falls. Luckily, no broken legs yet—knock on wood—but it is a constant concern. It is risky for me to leave Richard unattended for even one minute. That is exactly the minute he would pick to do some "fancy stepping."

If your dependent is mobile, don't keep throw rugs or small objects around that could be tripped over. The type of shoes your patient should wear depends a lot on the surface of the floor. Tennis shoes are more sure-footed on hardwood floors or when climbing stairs. A book I read said that leather soled shoes were better for patients with Parkinson's disease because of their tendency to drag their feet and freeze while walking. Rubber soles tend to catch on rugs, so I gave my husband's Reebok walking shoes to the Salvation Army. Well, I wish I had them back. A few weeks ago, while walking my husband across the wet back porch, those leather shoes slipped right out from under him. He fell and broke two ribs. With shoes, it's hard to know which type is most suitable. It makes sense to use the type that seems to work best for your patient on the floor coverings in your home.

A broken leg or hip would definitely add to your burden as a caregiver. Falls resulting in hip fractures are a common cause of hospitalization for elderly people.

Take care you don't break something yourself. That would be a double catastrophe. Hurrying won't get you anywhere, except into a plaster cast.

BUDGET your time and your money. They are equally important. I'm pretty good about handling time, but I come up short in the money department. I would revamp my budget, but it's vamped out. The minute I think there will be a sizable amount of money left over after paying bills, something big will break. It's just as sure to happen as death and taxes. I try to stick to a budget that's realistic and elastic because it always needs stretching.

Actually, I must confess, I should not try to tell anyone how to survive on a budget; I'm unqualified. I do know that savings should be put aside first because there is never anything left to save if it's the last consideration. I also know that you should pay off charge accounts in full each month, or cancel them. However, if you aren't able to pay the account off in full each month, make the effort to pay more than the minimum due. This will give you an excellent credit rating and at least decrease the amount of time it will take to clear the balance out. Having a credit card isn't all bad, though. Establishing good credit is important in this day and age for big purchases. It also saves having to carry a lot of cash with you. It is good to control spending. The deeper in debt you are, the deeper your worries.

Janice Hucknall Snyder

C

CALMNESS in a crisis is not always humanly possible, but when the unexpected happens, the calmer you manage to stay, the clearer your thinking will be. The opposite of calmness is panic. That is when thinking ceases completely and chaos takes over. To lessen the possibility of panic in a crisis, try preparing yourself in advance. Periodically, picture in your mind all the steps that you would take if: the house caught fire, your loved one started to choke or had a heart attack, someone was breaking into your home, or the toilet started to overflow. You don't have to be a scout to use the Boy Scout's motto: "Be prepared." When a plan has been formulated, there is a better chance that you will be able to stay calm and follow through in a crisis situation.

CARING shows in your eyes and in your touch. Even when the dependent is confused and unable to communicate with you, a hug or touch of the hand conveys that you care.

You don't have to qualify as disabled to need or receive a hug. Hugs are for anyone and everyone needing affection, which covers just about the entire human race. Hugs are one of the few things worth a million and cost nothing. If you are one of those people who don't like touching or being touched, give it just one more try. Go ahead. I hate to see you missing out on something that makes you feel so good and so cared about.

CAR REPAIRS are the pits, no pun intended. As if you didn't have enough to worry about, your car will be right there to test you further. It is important to keep the car running smoothly and safely. Are you one of those people who doesn't even know how to check the oil? If so, I surely do hope you know an honest mechanic to handle car problems for you.

Finding a good mechanic is a must, especially if the car is eight years old, like mine. You won't find "reasonably priced" auto repairs at a dealership. Ask around among your friends for an independent mechanic who is reliable. Preventive maintenance is an essential part of caring for your automobile and yourself. Regular check-ups can save a lot of aggravation, unplanned road stops, and perhaps even your life.

CHANGES get tougher the older you get. It is hard to change "set" ways. How well I know! This is another one of the difficulties you face when you suddenly find yourself looking after another person. There will be many changes in your life. Some changes will come suddenly, others slowly, but it is never-ending. There will be changes in the dependent's condition that require continuous accommodations and adjustments, which can be exasperating. Patience and flexibility are wonderful attributes to have when trying to get through these changes. Do not fret over the unchangeable; it's a waste of energy.

CHOICES are the decisions we all make, and a lot of them determine how our lives will be lived. Scary, isn't it? The easy, daily choices we make are what to eat, wear, and do for fun. Then, there are the big choices: your occupation, where to live, whom to marry, and the number of children to bring forth into this world.

Some choices determine your self-worth. When someone tries to intimidate you, it is your choice whether or not you allow it to happen. One of the ladies in my bridge club had been listening to a weekly TV program on psychiatry. One day she put what she had learned to the test. Over the card table, she told us how she had washed her husband's pants with his wallet still in them. When he got his soggy billfold back with the wet contents, he yelled in protest. Her response was to inform him of his responsibility to empty his pockets before placing clothes in the hamper. She said, "I don't blame you for being angry, but you screaming and hollering at me is unacceptable."

She chose not to be intimidated. She made a statement about her own self-worth, and in so doing, her husband gained awareness of and respect for her feelings. Using appropriate bridge terms, I would say she was "not vulnerable" to his intimidation and made a "grand slam." The rest of us were very impressed with her game plan. The choices you make not only affect your life but also the lives of others. Similarly, the decisions of others can affect you.

For the past ten years, I have worked with a patient who comes in every six months for an eye checkup. This 50-year-old lady, the youngest of eleven children, was born profoundly deaf. As a child, the whole family took care of her every need. They babied and spoiled her. Even though she was very intelligent, there was no incentive for her to learn sign language, so she didn't.

Janice Hucknall Snyder

This patient lives alone now and has a special phone and computer to help her communicate, but her behavior is still totally unacceptable. She screams sounds when she wants something. She slaps at people and makes faces when she isn't the center of attention. She is a very frustrated person. Her brothers and sisters can't stand to be around her now. Most of them have disappeared into the woodwork. Only one sister stood up to her and made her behave. Now this older sister has total responsibility for her care. She is the only one who can control her, or who cares to try. The sister has had a very rough time of it at that, and she is paying for everyone else's wrong choices. She is trapped in this unhappy situation.

Your task as a caregiver will be much easier if you make the right choices concerning your dependent's behavior from the very beginning. You will be dealing with frustrations and anger. You have a choice to make as to just how much unacceptable behavior you will allow. You control how things will be. As with a spoiled child, the more you let the dependent manipulate you, the more difficult it will be for you to control the dependent, especially later on. If your self-esteem is intact, you won't let the dependent take advantage of you.

Nobody likes to take orders. Give your dependent two choices in a given situation, but no more. If your loved one doesn't want to have a bath now, give the choice of in a half hour or an hour. This way your dependent retains some independence, which ups his/her self-esteem. Being firm and consistent, in a loving way, will help you to survive. It's your choice.

CHURCH attendance is not always practical after an illness or accident occurs with your loved one. If you have been an active member of a church and miss attending services, you do have some options. Perhaps you can get someone, or several people, to take turns staying with your dependent so you can attend services. Priests go to parishioner's homes to hear confessions and give communion to shut-ins. If your loved one stays in a day care center while you work, check with the nearest church of your denomination. It may be that the church offers a noontime service daily or once a week that you could attend on your lunch hour. If this is not feasible, there is always TV. Tune in to one of the many religious services that are broadcast. Choose one that is uplifting for you. Praying with the disabled person can be very meaningful and create a stronger bond between the two of you.

CLEANLINESS is next to Godliness. Proper hygiene is important as it promotes good health and good relationships. It is difficult to be around someone who has not seen the inside of a bathtub or shower recently.

Caregivers have the responsibility of maintaining the disabled person's cleanliness. It should be one of the top priorities in your already overloaded schedule. Good hygiene is especially important when the dependent becomes incontinent or immobile. Keeping the skin clean and dry prevents skin breakdown, thus decreasing the risk of infections. Changing clothes, bathing, brushing teeth and using deodorant should be done daily, or more if needed. When you control the bad smell, friends will ring your doorbell.

COMEDY, what would life be without it? Dull and boring, that's what. Life without the strains of laughter running through it would be depressing. Have you ever been around people who have no sense of humor? They take everything so seriously. They rarely smile and are not much fun at all.

Janice Hucknall Snyder

My husband and I have had situations where we didn't know whether to laugh or cry, like the time my husband came downstairs wearing one black and one brown shoe, with no socks. When I pointed it out, we looked at each other and burst out laughing. It looked so ridiculous, that was the only way to go.

When you get depressed, laughter is the medicine to get you back on track, and there are no bad side effects. Even when you are living in very serious, very sad circumstances, there is still room for humor and laughter. In fact, give humor all the room you can, it's one of the brightest spots in your life.

COMMITMENT to the person you are caring for goes without saying. When you find yourself in the number one position of caregiver, you are committed to doing all things for that person, twenty-four hours a day. Hopefully you have lots of family and friends willing to help with the caring in their free time. However, that is usually spasmodic, as most people do live busy, complicated lives.

Marriage is a serious commitment of two people sharing a life together. It is supporting each other through the laughter and the tears. When one of the marriage partners becomes totally disabled, that commitment is no longer shared. It becomes wholly and completely the caregiver's commitment. You miss having your partner's shoulder to lean on, help in managing the finances, and empathy, and you miss sharing each other's dreams. The reality is that one must be there for two, under the worst of circumstances. It takes a strong inner faith to keep that kind of commitment alive and well. It takes a very secure person believing that the power of love overcomes all. Without that belief, the caregiver would have a hard time keeping their commitment.

Survival of the Caregiver

If your disabled partner is cognizant, he or she has the added heartbreak of realizing his or her inability to contribute to the commitment and function as a normal helpmate. Your loved one has to watch, helplessly, while you deal with every aspect of survival. This can cause feelings of guilt, bitterness, and, subsequently, withdrawal unless a strong love is shared and communicated between the two of you.

COMMON SENSE is something I sure hope the good Lord gave you an ample supply of. Lord knows, as a caregiver, you need plenty. Common sense helps to get you through the problems of the day. Do use your common sense when it comes to keeping pills and poisonous liquids safely out of reach and having smoke alarms, adequate lighting indoors and out, and hand railings along all stairs. If your patient has some form of Dementia or Alzheimer's disease, you must "person proof" your house, just like you would child proof your home for a 2-year-old. Heavy things that could be grabbed or that can fall over on the patient should be screwed down or moved out of the way. Plants should be out of reach. I found my husband trying to eat the leaves on one. Sharp objects can be found in many areas. Do a room-by-room check, thinking, as you do this, about what things would be harmful to a young child, then clear them out. It will eliminate accidental injuries and save you a lot of grief.

COMMUNICATIONS between you and your dependent are important. Listen well. If the patient has trouble getting words out or making sense, try to find the words he or she is so desperately searching for. Check what is happening around the patient for clues. My husband, for example, will often pick up on what is being said on the TV and try to respond. Speak calmly and quietly, especially when the patient is in a state of agitation and frustration, and frustration there will be. Just imagine how you would feel if you were thinking something important and wanted to communicate it to someone, but the words coming out of your mouth made no sense at all, even to you.

The caregiver can get almost as frustrated as the dependent when attempting to interpret what is being said. Comprehension may fall short of the mark, but the times when you do get through to your loved one make the effort all worthwhile.

COMPARTMENTS in your mind prevent overload. When there are too many problems coming at you all at once, store some of them away for a while. It takes some practice, but it works. Usually, you will find solutions faster by using this method. Many people take their work problems home with them and fret over them all night. When I walk out the office door, any problems of that day are quickly dismissed. They are put away in a compartment and shut up tight. With a fresh mind in the morning, a resolution usually arrives quickly and easily. Try practicing compartmental thinking; you'll like how it can work for you. It isn't what happens to you but how you deal with it that makes the difference.

CONFRONTING the problems associated with being a caregiver boldly and squarely is the best way to go. There isn't time to do anything less. When problems occur, don't let them snowball. If you are having trouble handling your feelings, get them out or get help. If the patient is being irritable and difficult, confront him or her. Don't allow the patient to control you. That isn't a good situation for either of you. If some of the physical arrangements are difficult to handle, make changes that will ease the burden. Don't be afraid to ask for help. Don't be a martyr; a lot of martyrs died young.

COPIERS are valuable aides. I hope you have access to one. Many legal documents, such as insurance claims, doctor's reports, medication records, etc., need to be duplicated. Such records should be kept in your safe deposit box and filing cabinet respectively. Extra copies should be given to the appropriate people. Fortunately for me, there is a copier in my office. If one is not at your disposal and you need to use a copier often, buy a small, inexpensive version to do the job. In any case, there are copiers at the Post Office and certain stores that are available for a nominal fee. Although that is less convenient, it is still a good alternative. I promise you that sooner or later you will need to show proof of something that you or someone else have lost or misplaced. Duplications save a lot of wear and tear on the already stressed out you.

COPING is a word I don't like very much. The dictionary says it means to contend with a situation or problem successfully. Contend means to struggle with hardship and difficulty. So, then again, I guess it does apply to the caregiver's life, but I'd like to think there's a lot more to a caregiver's life than just coping—and there is, if you hold on to that good attitude I talked about under "A."

C.P.R. stands for Cardio-Pulmonary Resuscitation. It is vital for everyone to have knowledge of C.P.R. as you are then able to sustain life in an emergency situation. Courses in C.P.R. are offered in most communities. Don't put off learning this invaluable procedure; it saves lives. It would be terrible to have to stand by helplessly and watch a loved one in distress. If you have already taken the course, remember, it should be updated every two years.

Janice Hucknall Snyder

CREDIT is what you get when you sign an application form and are mailed one of those dangerous little plastic cards. I think it is important to have good credit and to keep it good. In an emergency, having a means to carry on is a necessity, e.g., if you run out of Depends with payday a week away. Help! Out comes the plastic. It is very easy to get in deep water with plastic credit, though. The key is to keep only one credit card and pay it off monthly. That's easier said than done and requires great self-control. As I've mentioned elsewhere, if you can't pay it all off, at least pay more than the minimum amount. Credit handled this way gives you excellent credit, less cost, and a lot less worry.

Shop around for your credit card company. I was paying 18.5% for years when I happened to watch a TV show discussing all the different types of cards and rates. They gave the address of a place that charged 8.5%. I wrote to that company immediately and have used them ever since. I get offers for new credit cards in the mail every month. They sound great, with all kinds of good deals and benefits, but read the fine print. The special rate may only be for the first six months, and the annual fee may be outrageous. Keep track of interest charges each month and add them up at the end of the year. You will probably be very unpleasantly surprised at how much it comes to.

CRUTCHES aid in walking, but those aren't the kind of crutches I'm referring to here. Many of us use unfortunate circumstances in our lives as crutches, or excuses, for our inability to perform in some way.

A favorite story of mine, which I told my fifth grade Sunday school class, was about identical twin brothers. At age eight, their mother died. The father was an alcoholic and unable to care for the children. Consequently, the twins were separated and raised by two different families. Thirty-five years later, they were located and reunited by a doctor studying twins. One twin was an alcoholic like his father; the other had never taken his first drink. When the alcoholic twin was asked why he became an alcoholic, he replied, "What else could I be, having a father who was a drunk."

When the other twin was asked why he had never taken a drink, he said, "How could I ever take a drink after seeing all the grief that my alcoholic father caused our family?"

One twin used his father as a crutch, an excuse, for his behavior. The other twin threw away that crutch and became his own person.

Each of us has these kinds of choices to make in our lives. Under the circumstances, caregivers could easily become bitter and unhappy. They could even justify feeling miserable or, in extreme cases, developing an addiction. It is not a very pleasant way to exist.

If you refuse to give in to the negative aspects of a situation, you will find there is no need for a crutch. Instead, you will discover many possibilities and opportunities for an enjoyable, meaningful life.

CRYING releases pent up feelings. When your emotions overflow but you don't want to upset your loved one, head for the shower. Have a good cry with the hot water pouring over you; feel yourself unwind as you let yourself go. Take slow, deep breaths until you're back together again.

It is important to handle tension before it gets the better of you. Learn to recognize the signs before stress becomes overwhelming. When I get impatient and start fussing about things, it's a clear signal for me to back off and give myself a break. Make sure you give yourself breaks, too. You deserve them!

D

DANCING is great exercise and a wonderful pastime. If you always loved dancing and now your partner's illness keeps you from this fun activity, try alternatives. There are places you can go to square dance or clog with a group. There are church dances, senior dances and even line dances. Give them all a try. Plan a night out at least once a month and kick up your heels.

Recently, I went to a Greek wedding. They have the right idea. Everyone gathered in a large circle. Holding hands, they circled around, doing various steps to the sounds of lively, delightful Greek music. What wonderful fun it is. I hope you've had the opportunity to go to at least one Greek wedding.

My mother loved to dance and was still dancing in her eighties. For years she refused to visit St. Petersburg, Florida. She said, "Everyone there is too old for me." (This comment was made when she was seventy-six.)

Finally, at age seventy-eight, she hopped on the train in Jacksonville, Florida and descended on that "old timer" city. She was in for a pleasant surprise. There were dances held nightly, and the "old fogies" were having the time of their lives. Needless to say, she danced every dance, every night, from then on. Mom often commented that she could have kicked herself for not going to St. Pete sooner. When she reached eighty-four, she decided she should stay closer to home, near our family, but this didn't stop her from dancing, oh no. Often, when I arrived at her home to spend the afternoon playing Canasta with her, I would hear one of her records playing. Tip-toeing up to the screen door, I'd stand quietly for several minutes, watching one spry ole gal dancing around the living room and singing to herself. It is one of my fondest memories. I often think of Mom when I'm dancing around the kitchen. Dancing will keep you young, so turn on the music and get those feet moving.

DAY-CARE CENTERS provide relief when it's needed the most. They also make it possible for the caregiver to continue full-time employment. The cost varies depending on the type of care given and the part of the country you live in. Ideally, the center needs to be close to your home for daily and weekend needs. The center should have a qualified nurse on duty at all times and one additional employee for every five clients. Check out the meals and activities provided. Drop in occasionally, if possible, to see how things are going. If your dependent is on Medicaid, it will help pay this expense.

DAYDREAMS are the things that give substance to your hopes and yearnings. Not all of them will come true, or are even meant to. But it is fun to use your imagination and escape for a while into the land of fantasy. Dreams take your mind off worrisome situations. As a child, I read a lot rather than watching TV. I think this helped me develop my imagination.

The imagination is a grand entity. Unfortunately, with all of the visual aids today, our imagination has been put out to pasture, which is too bad, so sad.

Dreaming is a form of visualizing. Keep on dreaming, for dreams can come true when you believe in them. In the meantime, they are great for sidetracking stress.

DEATH is a subject most of us would rather not consider as a possibility any time in the near future, but there's no getting around it. Sometimes death is shockingly sudden, other times it is the end result of a long drawn-out illness. As we all know, there are advantages and disadvantages to both ways. For this reason, it helps to always keep our relationships with each other wholesome and free from guilt.

When your loved one has a form of Alzheimer's disease, you perceive a gradual loss. Occasions of not being recognized by your loved one become more and more frequent. You never forget the first time that it happens, because it is an extremely heart-rending moment. For many years you've been close to this person and shared intimate feelings and experiences. Sharing is such a special part of any relationship. Now you are left with an aching void. You may actually find yourself grieving for the loss of your loved one long before they die, and you may feel very sad and very alone at times. One day, I realized that I was grieving. Although Richard is with me physically, the whole person, my dear hubby, has faded away before my eyes. Whenever he is clearer of mind he makes me laugh and tells me he loves me. These are very precious moments indeed, but they are poignant, too. It tugs at the heart to get a glimpse and brief reminder of how he once was. And yet, it's these same moments that help to fill the void I am feeling.

So, along with all the complications of caring for your loved one, you may be experiencing stages of grief. At first, you may not fully realize what is happening to you. After all, there is no body to bury and there are no funeral arrangements to finalize. This makes coming to terms with your loss even more difficult. Recognize the need to work through your anger and pain.

Grieving and death are a natural part of life, but so is living fully and joyously. Life is precious and tentative; don't waste a moment of it. Know that when this cycle of life moves on to a spiritual plane, healing will be complete, and there will be no pain or regret.

DEBTS have to be paid. One day, driving to work, I was waiting for the light to change when I noticed a bumper sticker on the car in front of me. It said, "I owe; I owe; so, off to work I go!" I had to laugh. Ain't that the truth?

Credit cards are an expensive way to spend money if you don't have enough to pay off the monthly balance, and a lot of us don't. As the costs of caring for the disabled increase, there will be fewer funds available for you to pay off your debts. This then adds the burden of higher interest rates. It's a vicious circle, and making ends meet becomes a constant worry. So, if you are getting deeper in debt, have the willpower and courage to cut up those credit cards. Free yourself of this stress. I still have two cards to go. My scissors refuse to open and close when they get near either of them.

DECISIONS can be tough to make. Some people are never able to make a decision. They change their minds many times over until you want to yell, "Do something, anything, even if it's wrong!"

There are many serious decisions that must be made during your loved one's illness. Major concerns, such as health matters and deciding on a nursing home, place a heavy burden on you, the caregiver. Other family members need to be involved in these issues. They can, however, have conflicting opinions that make the final decision even more difficult.

When making important decisions, first weigh all the options, pros and cons. Then discuss your concerns with the one person you feel is best qualified to help make the right decision, whether it is a doctor, psychiatrist, religious leader or other family member. We all know "too many cooks spoil the broth." Thus, too many "concerned" people involved in making a decision may cause dissension and chaos. The final decision should rest with you, the caregiver.

DEED TO THE HOUSE . . . where is it? Just make sure you know where it is and that you have access to it. The deed should be in your name only if the dependent is your husband or wife. Should the time come when nursing home care is a must and the monies are exhausted, Medicaid is a foreseeable solution. There is a thirty-day waiting period for a dependent to become eligible for Medicaid. You need to have full ownership of your house for a certain amount of time. Every state has different rules about this. It's best to check with a lawyer. If the house stays in your partner's name or both your names, at least half of the value of the house will go to Medicaid when you die. If there are children and grandchildren you wish to have inherit your estate, don't delay in changing the deed. There is more on this subject under "LAWYER."

DEHYDRATION can become a serious condition, requiring hospitalization in severe cases. If your dependent develops a virus involving diarrhea and vomiting and it goes unchecked for too long, dehydration will occur. If the patient's tongue feels dry, that is an indication that they are dehydrated. Keep giving the dependent lots of fluids such as Gatorade and apple juice. Get a prescription from the doctor for medication that will check the diarrhea if it will not interfere with the other medications being given. If your patient is unable to keep fluids down over several hours and is getting extremely weak, take him/her to the emergency room at the nearest hospital. The fluids can be restored with I.V. (Intravenous) infusion. If the patient cannot be moved, a visiting nurse should be called in. Recognize that it is better to seek help from professionals sooner rather than later. Don't hesitate to transfer some of the responsibility at such times. Besides, you need a break from time to time.

DEODORANT keeps your friends coming back. In this day and age, there is no excuse for body odor. In our office, we have a few patients who come in with serious body odor. We find ourselves hoping they won't need to be re-checked anytime soon.

Don't get careless, lazy or forgetful when it comes to hygiene. Daily bathing with soap, underarm deodorants and mouthwashes, will make life a lot more bearable for others in your dependent's life, and yours too.

DEPRESSION, in and of itself, is an insidious affliction that eats away at the very essence of man. It is a grievous illness that saps the will to live. The mental breakdown that can follow depression is a painful anguish to bear, and it is a heartbreaking experience for that person's loved ones. It is important for the caregiver to realize that suicide is always a possibility in cases with severe depression. Stay alert to that fact. If the patient starts to act a lot happier compared to usual, don't relax your vigil. Many times when the decision to commit suicide has been reached, the patient will seem better. The suicidal person feels relieved to know that the mental pain and anguish will soon be over.

When there is a debilitating illness, there is always a chance that it will be accompanied by depression. Recognizing and dealing with depression early on is imperative. You will not be qualified to deal with this problem if it is prolonged.

Consider finding a competent psychiatrist or psychologist to consult when help is needed. How do you go about this? Here are a few dos and don'ts. First of all, don't feel embarrassed or ashamed about your loved one's mental illness, because that is what it is, an illness. Do talk to other people. Even if they are not seeing a psychiatrist, they may know someone who is. Word of mouth can tell you a lot about a doctor's reputation. But don't expect a doctor who someone else thinks is just the greatest to necessarily be perfect for your loved one. You may have to search further if there is a conflict of personalities. Do ask one or two physicians you know for recommendations. Don't be influenced by the size of the ad in the yellow pages. Do make sure the doctor is Board Certified. Don't be afraid to ask the doctor questions; make a list. Do check with the local Medical Society to see if there are any complaints filed against the doctor you are considering. Don't put off finding someone suitable to treat your depressed loved one. Do get help now if it is needed. Don't let this become an, "If only I had. . ." kind of a situation.

Most communities have crisis prevention centers. Contact them for help and advice in dealing with depression. There are books in the library that deal with depression. They would be helpful reading for you, the caregiver, as well as the patient. Check them out.

Janice Hucknall Snyder

DIET is very important in the caregiver's stressful life. Eating the right foods keeps you physically fit. Good nutrition gives you the extra energy needed when caring for a loved one. Some people have a tendency to eat too much when under stress; others eat too little. Moderation in eating is best, with a splurge now and then, of course.

DISCIPLINE is a word you associate with the training of children, but it also has an important place in the caregiver's life. Discipline yourself to get things done in the order of priority. Otherwise, you'll find yourself up a creek in the management of your dependent. You'll lose out on time needed for yourself.

When you're tired, it's hard to make yourself write those checks or file that insurance, but what's put off has to be caught up. The longer you procrastinate, the harder it will be to straighten out the mess. This is especially so with insurance claims.

The way I discipline myself is to do the thing I like doing the least first. That would be ironing—a very pressing matter. Whatever I look forward to doing the most is in last place. That would be writing, reading or baking. With this routine, the incentive is great to get the yuckies out of the way quickly so I can get to the goodies faster. Discipline makes life easier and more productive, and it even provides extra time for fun and games.

DISCOMFORTS of the dependent can, hopefully, be treated effectively by a doctor. Don't ever hesitate to seek help in keeping your dependent free from pain. You and your loved one know best when that relief is needed. When the patient is feeling okay, so is the caregiver.

DISCOURAGED with the way things are going? That feeling can creep in at any time. When you have been dealing with your loved one's condition year after year, and the caring becomes harder and harder, it does get discouraging. When you take away the "dis" in discourage, what's left is courage. At times, courage is what keeps you going when disheartened. Courage is a strong ally to the caregiver.

DISRUPTIONS can be very disturbing to your schedule, and you need a schedule to survive. If disruptions are an occasional happening, going with the flow is the way to go. But if someone makes a habit of dropping in daily, especially when it's your personal time while the patient is napping, politely let the visitor know. Say that the patient has a regular nap period between 1:30 and 3:30 every day and shouldn't be disturbed during this time. Be polite, tactful and firm. Let visitors know what hours they are welcome to visit. A real friend will understand; all others are expendable. Sound severe? It's not if you want to survive.

DOUBT that you have the strength it takes to be a caregiver? Sure, many times you'll wonder how long you can keep up with the rigors of each day. When things are going badly and you're over-tired from lack of sleep, doubts will cross your mind. Keep them brief. Why? Doubts are on the negative side. There is no room in your life for those kinds of thoughts if you are to survive.

DRESSING another person is a different kind of challenge. How to handle the dressing depends on how much the disabled person can help you with it. No matter what, it is a task requiring fortitude. I find the hardest part of this "exercise" is allowing enough time to get the job done. It isn't something you can rush, and I say this with tongue in cheek. It helps to lay out clothes the night before. To save my back, I sit beside my husband on the bed. I put on his shirt and button it. Next, I lift the leg that is farthest from me, over my leg. I put the sock, pant leg and shoe (using a shoe horn) on that leg and repeat the procedure on the leg nearest me. Standing him up, (with his hand holding the grip bar) I tuck in his shirt and fasten the Velcro strip on his pants. The task is completed with the least amount of bending and exertion possible. Streamlining routines that require exertion helps to conserve your stamina.

If your patient is a woman, simple one-piece dresses are the easiest to put on and the most comfortable. Pull-on pants with an elastic waistband, along with an over-blouse does well too.

DROOLING is an uncontrollable, unpleasant and unattractive condition in some patients. If your dependent develops this problem, putting on a bib helps keep their clothing from getting saturated. Keep a tissue handy to blot the chin, especially when others are present.

DUTY is something you feel you ought to do or must do. It is a moral obligation, but it is not always something you would do if you had your druthers. I'm sure there are many people who take care of another person out of a sense of duty. When that is the case, accepting the responsibility is, emotionally, more difficult. Being a caregiver requires such dedication. When you have a loving relationship with the dependent, it eases the burden a great deal.

E

EFFICIENCY in your daily routine allows extra time for you. Just as pennies saved add up to dollars, minutes saved add up to hours.

If you live in a two-story house, keep such things as medications, diapers, shirts and pants on both levels to save trips up and down the stairs. When taking trips in the car, make a list of the stops and plan your route in the best order for saving time and gas. When shopping for paper goods and food, as mentioned under "BARGAINS," buy in large quantities. A freezer is a good investment. It enables you to stock up on the "specials" run by supermarkets. Efficiency saves you time, money and effort.

EMERGENCIES can happen anytime, anywhere, to anyone. Keeping a level head is important, but not always easy. Some people are able to stay calm, cool and collected. Others push the panic button fast. I do both. I panic first, and then I get calm and collected, but I am never cool.

If your dependent is bed-ridden, an intercom system in the house keeps you alert to any needs. There should be a plan if the house catches fire. If the dependent develops a serious medical problem or falls, be prepared. Keep a telephone on both floor levels, and keep the doctor's phone number handy, but call 911 first. Have a prepared list of the patient's medications, with the schedule and dosages given. Take it along to the hospital. Hopefully someone living close by can be called on to assist you until rescue arrives. Picture in your mind just what action you would take in an emergency. That will help you follow through should the need become a reality. See "CALMNESS" for more on this subject.

EMPATHY is the power to enter into the feelings or spirit of others. The patient needs a lot of empathy, but so do you. It helps to know someone who has experienced similar problems. That person can relate. Sometimes just the exchange of looks will say more than words and lift your spirits. This helps a lot at times when you don't feel like talking about what you are feeling.

Family and friends will say to me, "How are you doing?"

I could say, "Lousy," which may be the truth, but that's not what I want them to hear. More than likely, I will tell them that I'm doing just fine. Trying to be reassuring can get old though, month after month. But, then again, I'd be upset if nobody asked too. I think a great big hug is a wonderful substitute for words and expresses empathy in a very warm way. I hope you get lots of hugs.

EMOTIONS. Oh, yes, you have them, whether you admit it or not. Sadness? Yes, plenty of that. Anger? Lots of that, too. Shock? Every time things change for the worse. And grief for the loss of the wholeness of your loved one. You cannot survive if these are the predominate emotions in your life. If the burden of these feelings dwells in your heart most of the time, it will consume you; these feelings will break your heart and your spirit. When you offset sadness with joy, anger with calmness, shock with faith, and grief with acceptance, there will be peace in your heart. A sense of harmony gives you the ability to deal with all the possibilities of your life. If you believe in the power of prayer, praying for the strength to recognize and deal with negative emotions really does help.

ENCOURAGEMENT is something humans thrive on—caregivers, dependents or whoever. It is especially important for youngsters to get a good amount of encouragement in their formative years. Actually, we all need it, from the cradle to the grave. People are great at criticizing; how much more beneficial it would be if we gave encouragement instead. A pat on the back, along with a smile, doesn't cost a cent and is priceless to someone who is down and out. It gives caregivers a much-needed lift.

ENERGY is something you can't have too much of when you're a caregiver. Some people are born with extra energy. When kids are like that, we say they are hyperactive. Other individuals are very placid; nothing hurries them. I have a friend like that. A wedding shower was given for her, and it took her five minutes to open each gift. (I had to sit on my hands to keep from helping her.) She got some very beautiful things. Her monotone comment for each and every present was, "That's very nice. Thank you."

I wanted to shake her to see if it would get her motor running. My exclamations of delight far surpassed hers; you'd have thought the gifts were for me. As you may have surmised by now, I'm one of those over-energetic people. It's probably nice to be somewhere in-between, but inclined to the energetic side. Proper exercise, rest (try and get it) and diet are important. The right foods keep your motor purring smoothly so that you have that needed energy. Just as a car runs better when cared for, so does the human body. Sweets, around 2:30 in the afternoon, don't count though. I've convinced myself that a couple of pieces of fudge give me a much-needed burst of energy. Indulging yourself with candy is fine and dandy, as long as you take your vitamins and calcium and drink eight glasses of water a day first.

ENSURE is a dietary supplement that will help to sustain the patient who is losing weight. Hopefully it will even put some fat back on those bones. It can be bought in six packs or cases of twenty-four. Ensure comes in chocolate, strawberry and vanilla—all tasty flavors that are easy to drink. It is available in drug stores, grocery stores and places like K-Mart or Wal-Mart. Check around for the best price; it is expensive.

ENTERTAINMENT for you depends on the condition of your dependent. If the confinement is total, a DVD player brings movies and travelogues into your home. Cable TV has a great variety of shows too. If you enjoy games such as Bridge, Canasta, Poker, Backgammon and Dominoes, invite friends in for an evening of this kind of fun. Parlor games, like Monopoly, Scrabble, Pictionary, Boggle, Scattergories, and Trivial Pursuit, are entertaining and exercise the brain too.

If a good stage show is coming to town that you would love to see, don't be a martyr. Pick up that phone now and order tickets for you and a friend (collect their money later). Don't think it is unfair for you to have a night out on the town while your loved one has to stay at home. Go and enjoy. Let this be one of your times out when a "relief person" comes in. You deserve to have some distractions in your life, especially now that you have undertaken the continuing care of another. Diversion is needed if you are to keep healthy mentally, if you are to survive. Don't get so bogged down in your care of the dependent that you forget you have needs too. That is unhealthy. Unhealthy caregivers have less to give.

ENVY is not a good feeling. I don't know if other caregivers experience envy, but it has caught up with me at times. The phone will ring, and it will be dear old friends calling from six states away. It seems they will be passing through on their way to some lovely vacation spot to play tennis or golf. They just want to stop by and say hello. We are always happy to see these special people who have shared a part of our lives through the years. We look forward to their visits. But at such times, it really hits home hard that we'll never be able to do those kinds of "together" things again. I find myself envying their freedom to travel and do a variety of activities as a couple. It really hurts. At such times, I have to work a little harder at counting our many blessings. I have to remember to be thankful that we, too, were able to do many wonderful things before the illness.

Do you find yourself envying other's freedom? That feeling is understandable under the circumstances. Try to focus on the positive. Though your flexibility is limited, there are still activities you can enjoy doing. Make plans for the near and distant future. Having things to look forward to helps a lot when the present is restricted. The biggest limits are the ones we impose on ourselves with negative thinking.

ERRORS occur in everyone's lives. People have trouble admitting them for different reasons. For example, "perfect" people never make mistakes. Other people may fear retribution if they make a mistake, such as getting caught robbing a store. Still others may be embarrassed because their mistake was careless, or just a dumb thing to do.

Then there are those who make mistakes due to stress and fatigue, which would be you and I. I handle mistakes by apologizing, correcting them quickly when possible, analyzing why they happened and then putting them out of my mind. I hope you are able to do that too. You have enough problems to deal with without being down on yourself about mistakes.

EXAMINATIONS are something a lot of people put off and put off, some until it is too late. It's obvious why we don't like to go to the doctor. It's expensive, we're afraid they'll find something seriously wrong and it just isn't fun. But you have a responsibility to the dependent and yourself to take good care of your health. Fatigue, depression over your loved one's condition, financial worries and stress can each, on their own, cause illness in a caregiver. Be alert to the reality of this and have regular check-ups. Having to care for another when you are sick is not recommended. It's a nightmare. I know because I've survived it.

EXERCISE is another thing that gives you energy. "Oh," you say, "But by the time I get through with all I have to do, I don't have anything left to exercise."

Wrong. Remember how, when you were young, you would go to work all day and come home exhausted? And how then you would have a date that night? A quick hot shower and off you would go, dancing the night away. The same holds true with exercise. The secret is to find an exercise that you enjoy doing and can manage in your environment. If you are totally confined to the house, video exercises, weight lifting, and exercise machines can be fun. If you can get time away from the house, tennis, golf, jogging, walking, or swimming are marvelous exercises. I go to an Olympic size pool at a university nearby and swim laps as often as possible. At times, I catch myself saying, "I'm just too tired to swim today." Here's where discipline comes in handy. Usually I can talk myself into going because I know how important it is to my wellbeing. The amazing reality is that when you're finished with the exercise, you don't feel more tired, you feel exhilarated. You've gotten the ole circulation going and inhaled a lot of fresh oxygen. Best of all, exercise relaxes you and relieves stress, that alone makes it worth the effort. In a health bulletin I recently read, it said, "When the mind is tired, exercise the body. When the body is tired, exercise the mind." Keep in mind the importance of doing both to survive.

Exercise for the dependent depends on the mobility of the patient. There are varying degrees and types of exercises that he/she can do. The patient's doctor would know best which ones are beneficial for your loved one. If none have been suggested, ask. You can't go wrong giving massages or simply lifting and lowering limbs to keep muscles from tightening, shortening up, or even worse, atrophying. Whatever you do, it is better than nothing.

EXHAUSTION is exhausting. I'm not talking about your average, everyday exhaustion, but heavy-duty exhaustion. When you reach the point where you can hardly put one foot in front of the other and don't think you can go on another minute, it's time to call a time out. If you were a fortune teller, you could foresee when this point would be reached, like one week from Friday. Then you could go ahead and collapse on that date, because you would have somebody waiting in the wings to step in. But since you can't foresee the future, it's a good idea to plan for that eventuality. Do have a backup, someone who knows the ropes. Don't wait until you've collapsed on your face to call them. They might not be able to come right away. By the time they get to you, you might be too weak to get up and let them in. Plan some R&R, that's Rest and Relaxation. Take a break from your round-the-clock caring anytime you feel it's necessary for your survival. Hopefully there are other family members who can give a day of their time periodically, rotating turns. If not, it would be worth it to pay someone to come in, even if you could only afford a sitter for one or two hours. You owe it to yourself, as well as the patient, to take that break. Go for it. Incidentally, always keep a current list of medicines, dosages, and schedules posted in a conspicuous place for your relief person. Be sure you show your 'angel' where the medications and pertinent supplies are kept.

EXPERIENCE has always been my best, though toughest, teacher. Human beings are basically God's loving, caring creations. By the time you've grown up in a family atmosphere, chances are you've already experienced a lot of give and take, joy and disappointment. You've been cared for, and hopefully you've learned a great deal about caring for others. Therefore, when encountering problems, go with the flow.

Changes in routine or the patient's condition can be difficult. Experience gives you confidence in your ability to handle whatever comes your way. Experience eases the burden.

F

FACTS OF LIFE deal with reality. Death and taxes do happen. Taxes are predictable, but death usually is not. Our demise, or that of someone dear to us, is something we tend to pretend won't happen, at least not for many years. Dying is mysterious and frightening to think about because it separates us from all our loved ones. So we put our heads in the sand like an ostrich and block this part of life from our thoughts. Caregivers don't have the luxury of being like an ostrich, too much is at stake. This issue needs to be faced now, while the opportunity to do so is still here.

I cannot emphasize enough the need to get your affairs, as well as the dependent's, in order, especially if you are husband and wife. If the ill person's mind is beginning to be affected (developing Alzheimer's disease or another form of Dementia), it is most important to have that person sign a form giving you Power of Attorney while they are still able to comprehend what it means. Otherwise, you will not be able to handle that person's financial matters. You may not even be able to write a check. You are responsible for ensuring your own future by realistically looking ahead and considering all the possibilities. One of our patients was in recently for an eye check-up. Her husband had dropped dead three weeks before from a massive heart attack. She was still in mourning and shock. On top of all that, this poor lady was frantic because she knew her husband had an insurance policy somewhere in the house. She had spent days looking everywhere and still hadn't found it. I asked about a safe deposit box, but there wasn't one. Needless to say, she was in a terrible state. One day, the future will become the present. Be prepared.

FAIRNESS in the game of life is a mirage. Sadly enough, some children learn very early on that life isn't fair. Sooner or later, every individual has an unfortunate experience which makes him or her realize that fact. Some seem to get larger doses of unfairness than others. A lady brought her husband in for an eye examination recently. We started talking, and she remarked that the past year had been rough. I inquired further. She said her husband had a brain tumor removed, her father developed Alzheimer's disease, and her home burned to the ground. Life had certainly been unfair to her and her loved ones in a short period of time. I would have been devastated. This brave lady seemed to be holding up remarkably well.

Everyone gets some bitter with the sweet and has rough roads to travel. Just remember, there are a lot of bends in the road, and there could be a rainbow just around the corner. Try not to dwell on the unfair times. You need to keep hope in your heart, for there is always tomorrow. Each life has many turning points, and the next one may be the best ever. How do you know otherwise?

FAMILY should be the main support system for you, the caregiver. There are no words to express how much the emotional and physical support of our family has meant. We are very fortunate because all four of our married children live nearby—what a blessing that is. Their thoughtfulness and help go a long way to ease my burden. I hope you have a family and that they are close and caring.

Keep your relatives updated on the ill person's condition, so they know what to expect and how to relate. The personal contacts that your family make mean a great deal to the dependent, too. Visits from loved ones are the highlight of a long day.

As right as the above all sounds, the family is not always supportive. In fact, they can create conflict. They can be jealous and resent the time you have to spend with the disabled person. I was made aware of this recently. A patient told me about having to put her ninety-year-old mother, who suffered with Alzheimer's, in a nursing home. Her mother's erratic behavior and waking up at all hours of the night had totally exhausted her. She added that there had been a real problem with her husband, too. He felt neglected. It had reached the point that he would come and sit down next to her every time she was sitting by her mother. Even her daughter complained bitterly. She said she got little or no attention at all from her mother because her grandma was so demanding.

Keep priorities straight. Juggling your time to include all those you love isn't easy, but with forethought, it can be done. You can be so involved with the needs of the disabled that you don't realize other important people in your life are being overlooked. Stop once in a while and take stock. How does the rest of the family around you seem to be reacting to what's going on? If relationships become strained, you won't feel so good.

FEAR will eat away at your ability to function. I think the greatest fear I have, as a caregiver, is that something will happen to me so that I will be unable to care for my husband.

Some events in life are beyond our control. However, a lot of what we think and do is in our control. That is really what inspired this book. I feel strongly that we, as caregivers, can do a lot to minimize risks and fears.

Fear can be a debilitating factor in your life. The worst thing that fear does is prevent you from living your life fully and with zest. There are all kinds of phobias. All of them restrain people in some way. Phobias are a form of prison for the soul and spirit. Fear of failure keeps a lot of people from taking risks. The people who reach their goals of achievement have usually learned how to climb over their failures. You may fear the unknown, what the future holds and how you will be able to cope physically, mentally and financially. It is hard not to think about these things. All together they can be overwhelming. Turn fearful feelings over to God. It will help you have the courage to function well as a caregiver.

FEELINGS can be strong in the caregiver. You may have many bad ones, which fill you with shame and guilt. You won't even want to admit them to yourself, but they can rear their ugly heads when you least expect them to. The main thing to realize is that, as bad as those feelings and thoughts are, they are not abnormal. When you are enduring constant pressure and are "putting up with" annoying scenarios, it is normal to feel those kinds of emotions. I do wish I could be someplace else, far away without my loved one; I do get angry with him for taking my freedom away; I do dislike the unpleasant tasks I have to perform for him; I do feel unjustly put upon because he caused my life to be filled with his needs; yes, I do feel sorry for myself, and that's okay. I just don't let myself linger on those feelings for long periods of time. It helps to talk to an understanding person, someone you feel close to, so you can get those feelings out in the open. Then you can deal with them. When I've had a rough morning, getting my husband up, showered, dressed, shaved and fed, and getting bed sheets changed and washed, etc., I rush into the office with my spirits pretty low. Before long, a patient will come in whose problems put me to shame. I'm quickly over those "sorry for myself" feelings. I remind myself of how much I have to be thankful for. I concentrate on the many wonderful experiences my husband and I have shared and the beautiful people who are a part of my life—most especially the one I'm caring for. Accept the fact that you will have bad feelings. Deal with these emotions in a positive way. Then, you will be able to rise above them and feel good again.

FIRE is wonderful, in the fireplace on a cold winter evening with everyone sitting around roasting marshmallows and telling stories. But the thought of your house catching on fire is another story—terrifying. The difficulty of getting a disabled person out quickly and safely is obvious. Escape routes should be planned. A bedside phone is a must. Fire extinguishers should be on every floor level. Smoke alarms need to be strategically placed on the ceiling of every room and in every storage area. The city electric department will check out the house wiring when requested. Do not have over-loaded extension cords laying everywhere.

Things seem to keep happening that are giving me material for this book. I wish this particular one hadn't. Last week, our house could have actually burned down if we had been sleeping or out of the house. I smelled something acrid, which always gets the ole ticker beating faster.

Janice Hucknall Snyder

Glancing toward our closed in porch, I saw smoke curling up in the doorway. I raced out there and saw that an extension cord, which was laying on the rug, was smoldering. The lamp plugged into it wasn't even turned on. There was a hard-driving rain at the time. Water had seeped through the ceiling and was dripping right on the plug at the connection. It caused a near disaster. Scary, isn't it? I bought a bunch of smoke detectors the next day, deciding the one in the kitchen wasn't quite doing the job.

There are some things you can't do to prevent a fire, but everything you can do, should be done. Don't put off or neglect this important issue. Your local fire department is always happy to advise you on fire prevention and what to do in case of a fire. They are there for you. Give them a call. Make them aware of the fact that you have a disabled person in your home. Safety first, or sorry later.

FLOWERS are a joy to behold. Fresh flowers or plants add color and cheeriness to any room and are pleasing to the eye. It is a sentimental, loving gesture for a husband to give his wife a bouquet. Now that my husband isn't able to do anything like that, I do it for him. I usually succumb to this urge while in the grocery store, rationalizing that flowers are better for me than two boxes of fattening cookies. Works every time. Try treating yourself to a bouquet of pretty flowers once in a while. You'll find it is an inexpensive way to cheer yourself up.

FOOD can be a problem for the dependent with coordination problems. Cutting meat and other solids may become too difficult to handle. If you have guests, do the cutting before placing his/her plate on the table. It will save your loved one embarrassment. Place the meal in a curved dish to make the food easier to pick up. Serving finger foods, like chicken wings, pizza, corn on the cob and

French fries, works well too. Keep a plastic place mat under the plate to catch spillage and ease in clean up.

Once, a young man named Jimmy, along with his college buddies, had been chug-a-lugging from a keg of beer. Jimmy then dove into the surf and broke his neck. I lived nearby and saw his friends dragging him out of the ocean. I grabbed a blanket and ran down to the beach. As I covered him up, he told me he couldn't feel his legs. My heart sank. He did feel my hand holding his and kept saying, "Please don't let go."

I kept telling him he'd be all right, although I feared the worse. I visited Jimmy after his surgery at the rehabilitation center. He was very lucky. He was regaining feeling in his legs and arms and making great progress. Jimmy was feeding himself with great effort, but with pride at being able to do so. The nurse had tied a spoon to his hand, and the spoon was bent into a curve. That made it possible for him to maneuver the food to his mouth. More important, it gave Jimmy some needed independence, which was vital at that point in his recovery.

Jimmy came by my office a couple of months later. He told me he was returning to college. He still used a cane, but he wore a big smile on his face. I was smiling too. It was a happy ending for someone who came close to being a quadriplegic.

There are ways to adapt utensils and dishes so your dependent can function alone. Any aide that helps grant independence in any activity is crucial for the self-esteem of your loved one. Anything that makes the dependent feel better makes you feel better too.

FORCEFULNESS may seem like a drastic action, but there are times when it is imperative that the caregiver be forceful with the patient. When the patient's safety is at risk, you must stand your ground. This can be difficult for wives who have always been totally dependent and submissive to their husbands. That isn't the case in my marriage, but it can still be a dilemma. My husband always used a regular razor. When he developed coordination problems, he got so he was cutting himself daily. He stubbornly refused to switch to an electric razor. His reason being that it wouldn't shave him as well. Change is difficult for all of us. I asked, "How about growing a beard?"

He didn't want that either. Instead, I had one of the children give him an electric razor for Christmas, and at the same time, all the disposable razors managed to disappear. Needless to say, after using the new method of shaving for a while, he decided it was okay. I didn't miss seeing his cut up, bleeding face every morning at breakfast at all. Now that I have to shave him, I am doubly glad I was forceful back then. If there are changes that need to be made for the benefit of your loved one, your judgment must prevail.

FORGIVENESS works two ways. You need to be able to forgive others for the hurts they inflict upon you, and you need to ask and accept forgiveness for your unkind words and deeds. If this sounds a little familiar to you, it is because it's similar to a portion of The Lord's Prayer, "Forgive us our trespasses, as we forgive those who trespass against us." That is a very powerful statement. Too often we mouth the words but don't follow through on them.

When you are unable to forgive another for hurting you, you create a separation. The ones you love the most are the very ones who can hurt you the most. It is sad to hear about family members who haven't spoken in years. Should one of them die, the opportunity for forgiveness is gone forever.

Many people hold grudges. I know a person who, given the chance, will tell you, in detail, all the hurtful things other people have done to her over the last sixty-five years. What unhappy thoughts she holds "dear." The hardest thing of all can be forgiving yourself. I'm sure you've heard someone say, "I'll never forgive myself for that."

Never is a very long time to be down on yourself. No one should put that burden on himself or herself. Do not judge others, and try not to judge yourself. I have yet to meet a perfect human being: one who has never made a mistake or hurt another person. All cannot possibly be perfect in your relationship with your dependent every minute of every day. When needed, find forgiveness in your heart for the both of you.

FREEDOM is a precious gift. Appreciate it. I asked a patient about his wife, whom I knew had been suffering from Alzheimer's disease for five years. He said, "I can't afford to put her into a nursing home, and she requires care twenty-four hours a day. She doesn't sleep most of the night, so I catch naps when I can. You know, someday I hope I'll be free to go anywhere I want. That would be so wonderful." He had a poignant, little boy smile on his tired face. My heart went out to this seventy-eight-year-old man. I couldn't help but think that his freedom may only come through his own death, while his wife remains in her living death. It is truly a tragedy.

Your freedom to come and go is taken for granted and never really appreciated until you've lost it, and then how much it is missed! Situations beyond your control can and do take away your freedom. You cannot change that. However, how you react to what happens is your choice to make. If you react in an optimistic way, you can survive.

Janice Hucknall Snyder

FRIENDS are a blessing. Since a caregiver's time for socializing is restricted, you tend to narrow your relationships to just your very closest and dearest friends.

My husband's ability to communicate has become more and more limited. A lot of times, the words he thinks he is speaking are not what come out at all. This, plus problems with walking, have made attending gatherings uncomfortable for him. When we are with a few of our intimate friends, he's more at ease and even kids about himself. They, in turn, know what to expect. They are patient, caring and loving, listening and responding to whatever Richard is saying, no matter how senseless. These friends are truly treasured in my heart.

FRUSTRATIONS are something the caregiver deals with daily. There are plenty of little aggravating things just waiting to happen. My biggest frustration comes from the smallest thing: the remote control for the TV. Where is it? It does a disappearing act at least once a day. I've found it in every room of the house, upstairs and down, in pockets, in the bookcase, in waste paper baskets, you name it. People will say, "I can handle the big problems. It's the little ones that get to me." Well, this little one sure does get to me. Having to take time to look for things is not my favorite thing to do. It truly is frustrating.

On the serious side, it is frustrating to watch your loved one struggling to do something. If I am in a hurry, which I am a lot, I'm tempted to take over and do things for him. I know I shouldn't, but I don't always win that battle with myself.

When the dependent gets frustrated and there is difficulty communicating, that frustration can rapidly turn into agitation and anger. This becomes a more serious problem.

Survival of the Caregiver

The first time it happened to me, it was a shock (my husband had always been such a gentle person, never even raising his voice). I stayed calm, but it didn't help. After several minutes of loud screaming, (which seemed much longer) his anger subsided. Actually, it was probably good for him to get his feelings out. Maybe I'll try having some yelling sessions for 'fun.' Releasing tension is what it's all about.

If your dependent becomes more and more agitated, to the point of getting physical, then there are appropriate drugs with calming effects that should be given.

FUN belongs in the caregiver's daily schedule. Don't go to bed without having had some. Granted, being a caregiver is a serious responsibility and a wearing ordeal, mentally and physically. That is all the more reason why you should have something to do that is fun. It doesn't have to be a big deal. Make a list of a variety of things that are enjoyable to you, and depending on the daily circumstances, pick one that is suitable for the time you have. Be creative. See "HOBBIES."

FUTURE happenings can only be imagined. You don't know what the future holds; do you? Live each day to the fullest, and be thankful for it. Worrying about your future does not one bit of good. Plus, it could increase your blood pressure and stress, two things you don't need.

Janice Hucknall Snyder

G

GENTLENESS is the attribute of a patient soul. One of the things that your dependent needs the most is your gentleness. When caregivers are over-tired from over-caring, they get impatient. Impatience can turn into anger. Sometimes that anger is taken out on the patient. When that happens, there is no gentleness in your voice, your words or your actions.

I am very human, and as such, I have a "few" human frailties. I experience fatigue at times. Yes, and I have had "ungentle" moments with my loved one. I regretted each and every one of them. It is not easy to share my negative behavior with you. I do so to point out that even loving caregivers have limits of tolerance. You need to recognize what is happening in these types of situations. It is not unusual to become so stressed out that your behavior becomes less than gentle. It is a known fact that some caregivers go so far as to totally neglect their dependents, even deserting them. Through recognizing your limits, you can control the problem and limit unpleasant occurrences. When you find yourself yelling and losing your temper, it should be a warning signal to you. It's time for some of that R&R. Even a short break and change of scenery does a world of good to get things back in perspective.

If that isn't possible, to a hot shower or a soak in the tub you go. Or, head to a quiet corner in your home for fifteen minutes of meditation. Most important, be aware that you need to do something quick to defuse the situation. Then do it. You'll feel a whole lot better, and so will your dependent, who caused your frustration in the first place.

GIVE AND TAKE is what goes on between two caregivers. You probably already know some caregivers and will meet more. They are not hard to find. Caregivers have a lot in common, so we can be understanding listeners for each other. It helps when you can relate to one another's needs and emotional concerns. I always get back as much or more than I give. Spouting off can be great therapy. Check your local newspaper for the meeting schedule of a group that would best relate to the problems you have in caring for your dependent. Then give it a try—just one visit. That is the only way you will find out if this type of sharing therapy is for you.

GOALS for the dependent will depend on the area and degree of disability. Some patients can be rehabilitated. They are able to re-learn certain skills. They can have realistic goals to reach for. Hope, prayer, faith and determination add up to inner strength, which can even prove doctors wrong. I've seen patients that have beaten all the odds. It does happen, so do miracles. I pray with my husband every night at bedtime; it makes us both feel better. It's a nice, peaceful way to end what otherwise may have been a day of aggravations. If you are not comfortable with doing something like this, that's okay too.

The caregiver should always have lots of goals to reach for. Goals give one a sense of continuance, something to look forward to. One's self-esteem stays alive and well when achievements are reached. How many goals are you working on right now?

GRIEF for the loss of a loved one has no time limit, from beginning to end. It does not always begin at the time when the loved one is pronounced dead.

When a partner commits adultery, the husband or wife experiences grief for the loss of trust. In a divorce, one or both parties feel grief for the loss of companionship and the failure to sustain a loving relationship. The caregiver grieves for the loved one who is suffering and is so helpless. The family of a person with Alzheimer's grieves over the gradual loss of their loved one's recognition and ability to communicate. In all of the above cases, there is also grief for the loss of what might have been.

Each person grieves in his/her own way and for as long as he/she needs. Acceptance and getting on with life can only come when the person grieving is ready to let it. Some people need to hold on to grief because it is all they have left of a person. Certain people need the sympathy and attention that they get from others as long as they grieve. Still others never accept the loss of their loved one. I heard a man on TV say that he had never accepted the death of his son. In his mind's eye, he still pictured him alive, living someplace else and working as an architect. Grieving is a very personal thing. When and how long you choose to grieve should never need to be justified. Healing is helped along by getting involved in outside activities and helping others.

GRIP-BARS have holding power for your dependent. Strategically located, they provide stability and prevent falls. If your loved one has a problem maintaining balance, as in Parkinson's or a stroke, the bars will give the patient a feeling of security. I put one by the bathtub to aid my husband when getting in and out. Other grip-bars are by the toilet and bed. They help him to pull up and stand steady. When he is gripping the bar, it frees both of my hands to do other things for him. Grip-bars can be purchased at any hardware store. They are inexpensive, easy to install and well worth it.

GRATEFUL for your lot in life? You say, "What's there to be grateful for?" The answer is, "plenty." No matter how bad things are, they could always be worse. Really, I know there are times when that is hard to believe.

When all else is looking very bleak, I still have our family and friends to be grateful for. I hope this is true for you too. When you are submerged in the negative aspects of your life, it is hard to come up with anything to be grateful for. You tend to lose track of the positive things, past and present. Stop and think about this. Then sit down and make a list of all the things you are grateful for. I think you will be surprised at how long the list will get, and how much better you will feel.

GROWING is what life is all about. If you don't use it, you lose it. This is not just a cute saying; it is a fact. The saying usually refers to the physical parts of your body, but it is also true of your mental capacity. It is important to keep communication lines open in your brain. Keep your mind stimulated with mental exercises not found on TV. Take home courses, diversify your reading, play word games, write, etc. Stir up that grey matter.

The need to grow is also true for the disabled. Crippled bodies do not mean crippled brains. Challenging thinking activities can be a great morale booster. Your encouragement will help to get a response and raise your loved one's spirits. When the mind is concentrating on learning, it hasn't time to think about the negatives. This will benefit you both.

GUILT enters our lives sooner or later—usually sooner. Almost from the time we are born we are made to feel guilty about all sorts of things. Parents are experts at putting "guilt trips" on their children, and so the cycle goes round and round. Guilt eats away at your happiness. It is a miserable feeling. So if you have any guilty feelings, grit your teeth, own up and do what it takes to get this monkey off your back. Ask forgiveness of the offended person, or seek absolution through your religion. Do something to counteract the wrong and to show your sincerity. Take corrective actions before the guilt affects your mental as well as physical health. Guilt is a heavy load to carry. Lighten up!

Janice Hucknall Snyder

H

HABITS are formed early on; they are difficult to break. Just try! My parents tried several methods to break me from sucking my thumb. They put bitter-tasting medicine on my thumb at bedtime, sewed up my pajama sleeves and tied a form-fitting metal brace over my thumb. I suffered the bitterness, took off my pajama top and worked on the knot in the string for however long it took to get it untied. I quit when I was good and ready, and my reward was braces. It takes a great deal of willpower to stop a bad habit. If it is something that affects your health, like overeating or smoking (even affecting others around you), that should be incentive enough. Put your willpower into action. Replace bad habits with good ones. You can do it, one day at a time.

HAMSTRINGS are one of the five tendons of the thigh muscles behind the knee. You use them or lose them. When the dependent's ability to walk becomes difficult, as with Parkinson's, these tendons tend to tighten and draw up from lack of use. When this happens, walking is out and the wheelchair is in. Stretching the hamstrings helps to postpone that inevitability. While the dependent is sitting or lying down, lift each leg up as far as you can. Try to keep the knee from bending. Do this exercise ten times on each leg at least once or twice a day. It is hard work, but pushing a wheelchair and loading it into the trunk of your car is even harder.

HAPPINESS for one man could be another man's unhappiness. But one thing's for sure, if someone you love has a devastating illness, it is going to affect your happiness. Your life, for the most part, is dealing with what can only be perceived as an unhappy situation. It is most important that you retain your capacity for happiness. If your dependent is in a state of depression, that doesn't mean you have to mirror those feelings. On the contrary, you need as much happiness as you can get. It will help to keep up your spirits and the dependent's. Don't be one of those people who say, "It wouldn't be right for me to have any fun or happiness with my loved one so ill." And for heaven's sake, don't feel guilty if you get to enjoy an outing. Each life should be lived to capacity, so don't leave yourself out.

HEALTH of the dependent is the caregiver's constant concern. Often your loved one requires so much attention that you neglect your own health. This could lead to a critical situation should you become seriously ill. It puts a double burden on others. Get enough rest, eat properly, exercise and have regular check-ups with the doctor and dentist. For your mental health, be sure to set aside enough time for enjoyable activities. You have a better chance of surviving when you take good care of yourself. Your family will be grateful too. In fact, they will be ecstatic that they don't have to be caregivers for two.

HELPLESSNESS is devastating. When an independent person becomes totally dependent on another, it has to create a feeling that is positively frightening. Mental as well as physical support from you, helps to alleviate that sense of helplessness. The more calm and self-assured a picture you present, the more secure the distressed patient will feel with your management.

You, the caregiver, may also feel a sense of helplessness, with just cause. Your loved one has an incurable illness. All your efforts will not prevent the condition from deteriorating. You are helpless to change what cannot be changed. Watching this happen causes deep sorrow. When those feelings close in on me, it's time, once again, to count my blessings. (I do a lot of counting.) Don't let feelings of helplessness consume you. They are strong feelings that can do you in. Beware! Remember, when one door closes, another door opens, so never give up.

HOBBIES are something I hope you have plenty of. If not, start now to find one you can enjoy. A lot will depend on your financial situation. Your hobby can be as simple as reading, doing crossword or jigsaw puzzles, handwork, gardening, collecting things or even just jotting down your thoughts. More expensive and complex hobbies would be woodworking, stained glass, photography, painting, stamp collecting, computer games; you name it. Have at least one hobby. In fact, try several. The more the better. Don't be concerned about not having a special talent for your hobby. That's not at all important. A hobby is supposed to be something you do for fun. Don't put pressure on yourself of having to do it perfectly. That defeats the whole purpose. The objective is to have a much-needed outlet, a release from the pressures of being a caregiver. The best kind of hobbies involve your total concentration.

Take time each day for your hobbies, even if it's only for fifteen minutes. Hobbies are a wonderful escape, and they are good for keeping your sanity too.

HOPE, without it, all is lost. The word hope represents life itself. When someone who is ill is in a life-threatening situation, struggling to survive, and he or she loses the will to live, they will die because they have given up hope. When you have a deep faith, hope is its companion, and it helps you to stay strong. Hope is what gets you through the rough times. It is what helps you to survive. That one word holds so much power. It is truly incredible.

A line in one of Roger Whitaker's songs goes, "And I can see the new tomorrow coming on." The main theme of the song is that tomorrow never comes, that you should live for today. This is my philosophy too. But that one line expresses the hope that life is renewed each day and there are new tomorrows coming. Never forget that discoveries of new cures and breakthroughs in diseases are happening all the time.

Caregivers and patients should never stop hoping for what is best in any given situation. Hope can sustain you and the ill person. Hope can get you through to a better time, as long as you keep your heart and mind filled with it. Hope, along with faith, has an uplifting power. They go hand in hand in the healing process.

HOSPICE is an agency that provides support and care for people in the final stages of life, and for their family. I have never needed their services, but I know many people who have. I've been told that along with all the special caring, they do such things as making arrangements for hospital admission and filling out insurance claims for you. I have heard nothing but accolades for the Hospice program. Initially, a doctor prescribes Hospice when he or she feels a person has approximately six months to live. I recommend looking into what they offer when your loved one reaches a time when it would be beneficial, for all concerned, to have their comforting care.

HOLDING AND HUGGING, wow, is this important. I put these two words together because they are similar, but there is a difference. A hug is more of a quick, affectionate embrace. Holding is much longer, with deeper feeling. It's a transfer of warmth and love between one another. I love to do both. Hug and hold often. This interaction says a lot more than words. Holding is especially meaningful at times when words are difficult to express, or inadequate. I hope you practice hugging and holding a lot with your loved one. Practice makes perfect, and both of these H words are perfectly good for you.

Janice Hucknall Snyder

I

ICE CREAM goes down easy and is yummy for the tummy. Homemade lemon ice cream is divine. In case you have an electric ice cream maker and want to try it, here's the recipe:

10 lemons
1 (12 ounce) can of evaporated milk
2 quarts of Half and Half
3 cups sugar
1/2 pint of whipping cream

Grate 5 lemons. (This is the hard part, but it is still worth it.) Squeeze the juice from all 10 lemons. Combine lemon rind and juice with all the other ingredients in the container that comes with your electric ice cream maker.

When the machine has finished making the ice cream, place the soft ice cream in plastic containers in your freezer if there is any left after everyone has tried it. I have made it and just poured it into a Tupperware container and put it in the freezer without using an electric mixer at all. It is a lot less work and still tastes very good.

Ice cream is very nourishing and a delicious treat. Unless your patient is not supposed to eat ice cream for some particular reason, serve it often. This dessert is good for the patient who is on the thin side and is easy to eat for those who have trouble swallowing. I add a lot of ice cream to milk shakes for my husband. He loves them. Substitute yogurt if you prefer. And don't forget to make the lemon ice cream; you'll be glad you did.

I.D. BRACELETS can save your dependent's life. If the dependent is ambulatory, he/she needs to wear one. The bracelet should show the person's name, address, phone number, illness and drugs needed. A diabetic in a coma could mistakenly be considered drunk. It has happened. That could prove to be fatal.

A person with Alzheimer's disease could wander off, bewildered and lost. My husband slipped out of the house one time. It was a frightening experience. The only comforting thought I had, while frantically running here and there, screaming his name, was, "Thank God, he's wearing his bracelet."

I found him standing at our neighbor's back door, looking quite unconcerned. He couldn't understand what all the fuss was about.

You can purchase I.D. bracelets on the Internet. Go online and you will find several places to buy them and have them engraved.

ILLNESSES that the caregiver develops are a downer. If you do get sick with a bad cold, severe headache, virus, back strain, or you name it, keep smiling, even though your eyes are bleary and your body's wracked with pain. Am I making you sound like a martyr? Well, you are. And yes, there are times when the caregiver could use some sympathy too. However, when I'm not feeling good and it shows, I usually wish it didn't.

Dependent people have a difficult time dealing with their caregiver being ill. They feel like more of a burden, more vulnerable and more anxious. Nevertheless, I have been known to moan and groan at times. Have you ever tried buttoning someone's shirt with dry, cracked fingertips? Ouch! When you have your hands in water a lot, keep the hand lotion handy. Keep a stiff upper lip too.

IMPATIENCE can take hold of you more often than you'd like to admit. When I'm on a tight schedule, which is most of the time, and there are "incidents" to throw it out of whack, I could scream. And I do! That's okay. You've got to let it out sometime, and sooner is better. Built up steam makes a bigger explosion. My impatience can rear its ugly head when my husband spills something during a meal; it usually goes all over the food or all over his clothes, which then need changing. To top it off, we're probably already late for an appointment. It's just another one of those times when taking slow, deep breaths and counting to 100 helps. Patience is a virtue; being a caregiver sure puts it to the test.

INDIVIDUALITY makes you special. You are you and nobody else. The expression "comparisons are odious" is very true. Keep that in mind when some well-intentioned person starts telling you how they think you should be handling your situation. You might hear something like, "Well, Betty has similar problems caring for her father, and she handles that procedure differently. I just know it would be easier if you did it that way too."

Listen to advice, because some of it can be very helpful, but don't feel you have to go along with it or explain why you won't. What works for another person might not be comfortable or right for you. Keep an open mind, but hold your own counsel. Your judgment must prevail. Don't let a persistent "know it all" intimidate you. In fact, don't let one get near you. The last thing you need is to have your confidence as a caregiver undermined. Remember, nobody can make you feel inferior about anything you're doing without your permission.

INSURANCE is a living nightmare for the caregiver. Be thankful if your dependent is covered by one or two policies. When several doctors are caring for the ill person, the only way to keep it straight is to make up a chart. Have columns for the doctor's names, appointment dates, charges, when filed, when paid by each insurance company, deductibles, co-payments met, etc. (See my insurance spreadsheet at back of book.) Keep a separate chart for hospital charges. Try not to pull your hair out while doing all of the above.

My husband was in the hospital for three weeks. A month later, I got a huge bill of thousands of dollars from the doctor involved. That is when I made my first chart. It took me a whole weekend, working several hours each day, to get order out of chaos. Then I still had to straighten out the insurance department in the doctor's office. You may have already figured this out by now, but not all personnel in doctors' offices are insurance experts; big mistakes do get made. I got the bill resolved. I owed nothing.

Working in a doctor's office for many years has made me knowledgeable about insurance. But for the average person, the ins and outs of insurance can be very confusing, in which case you are out of luck, and a lot of money besides. Many people pay bills they don't really owe, or they go ahead and pay when the first bill comes. Wait until you receive the doctor's statement showing the payment from the insurance company. If your patient is on Medicare and the doctor "accepts assignment," the statement should also show that the non-allowed amount has been written off. Now you can pay the balance, unless you have a second insurance. In that case, you probably owe nothing if you have met your deductible. It is imperative to keep accurate and up-to-date records when you are caring for someone with a catastrophic illness. It makes good sense and saves money.

Statements for hospital charges should be checked closely too. Even though the hospital files directly to the insurance company, go over each item on your bill for errors. There was a special featured on TV about erroneous hospital charges. One lady had a bill showing a charge of over $300.00 for seven sticks of gum. Another charge was for something she didn't receive at all. Don't hesitate to call the hospital business office about any charges in question. You and your insurance company deserve an answer.

A word on other types of insurance, if your dependent was in charge of paying the Homeowner's, Automobile, Health and Life Insurance, you need to take over this responsibility now. Married couples should communicate with each other on these matters from day one of their marriage. Both parties should know where all the necessary papers are at all times. When a person has a stroke, communication can be lost. Do you know how the mortgage and taxes are paid? When are the insurance payments due? Where are the policies? Do you have access to the safe deposit box? Are the deed to the house and your wills in there? Checking these types of things out is something a lot of people put off and put off until it is too late. Will you be too late?

Don't make the mistake of allowing your spouse to have total and complete charge of important records. If or when bad news happens, you will have enough to worry about. You don't need the added stress of searching for documents. Be prepared.

INTERCOMS are an essential item to have in your home, especially if you live in a two-story house. They help you keep tabs on your dependent upstairs while you are downstairs. You save a lot of steps by not having to run up and down to check.

The ill person, who is usually sleeping in a separate bedroom, needs monitoring during the night. I'm a heavy sleeper and would be lost without this wonderful device. I sleep much better knowing my husband doesn't have to yell his lungs out to get me to hear him at 2 a.m. Intercoms are available in many stores and on the Internet.

INTERCOURSE is a very personal subject, but it has a place in this book too. When it comes to intercourse, one healthy caregiver plus one dependent partner can equal a fond memory. When lost, this intimate, most natural and fantastic part of a loving relationship in marriage becomes just a memory. Depending on the circumstances of the illness, intercourse may cease suddenly or gradually until, eventually, completely. For a great, new and current solution, check the section on Viagra under "V."

There are several drugs that cause impotence, even in people who are not incapacitated. A big, strong man came into our office very upset. It seemed the eye drops another doctor had prescribed for him was causing him to be impotent. Now who would think eye drops could do that? But certain ones can. Doctors don't always tell a patient about the side effects of drugs they prescribe. The power of suggestion can increase the likelihood of the patient experiencing the side effects.

Drugs are an essential part of an ill person's survival and comfort. They are also what I call a necessary evil because there can be many serious side effects. Parkinson's disease can be drug related. I fully believe my husband developed Parkinson's as a result of taking drugs for depression over a period of many years, drugs that also made him impotent.

So what's a healthy caregiver to do if the disabled person is his/her marriage partner? Find an outside interest? Some people can do this, but I feel it's not proper when you are committed in marriage. Corny as it may sound in these times, when you truly love someone, you don't run around on him or her. You took him or her for better or worse, in sickness and in health, remember?

Also, there is the added inconvenience of contracting the AIDS virus now. That's not a lovely thought to a caregiver, whose good health is so essential to the dependent's every comfort and very existence. So, the obvious solution requires me to use a word that many people find offensive and distasteful. Why? I don't know, because it is not really such an unnatural act. The word, as you may have guessed, is masturbation. I would rather call it self-gratification. If you have enjoyed an active sex life in your marriage and this is taken away by unnatural circumstances, whether you are forty or seventy, a very important part of your being is now lacking or entirely missing. So, self-gratification is not only a viable solution, it is essential to your continued good health and survival.

Most important, besides being pleasurable, the act itself is a very significant means of releasing tension. If there is one thing a caregiver has plenty of, it's tension that needs releasing. I cannot stress enough how healthy "relieving stress" is in your life. It keeps you balanced. It gives you the ability to deal with all the nitty-gritty problems, without losing control yourself. On the plus side, with self-gratification, you get to choose when. There is never a need to say, "Not tonight dear, I have a headache."

J

JARGON is defined in the dictionary as confused, unintelligible talk. If your dependent has Alzheimer's or other forms of Dementia, you know all about jargon. It is such an agonizing thing to see someone you love, who is highly intelligent, struggling to speak the words he or she is thinking. The words may be spoken as a mass of unassociated utterances. The saddest part is that the person speaking this gobbly-gook hears what is being said and realizes it isn't what he or she is trying to communicate. How frustrating is that? No wonder they have angry outbursts.

When the words aren't coming out right, I listen carefully and try to get the gist of what is meant. Sometimes, it is an effort to comment on what we are doing or saying at the time. Pointing to things and prompting can attain comprehension. The ability to relate becomes more infrequent as the disease progresses. This problem is also frustrating for the caregiver trying to decipher what the loved one may be asking for. Patience is indeed a virtue at such times.

JEOPARDY may be a factor in the life of your patient. The patient with Alzheimer's disease must be protected from hazards or his/her life could be in peril. The need for precaution is very evident in the mobile person who is childlike. It requires constant alertness on your part. Things that can be dangerous, such as matches, pills, sharp objects, poisonous liquids, etc., should be kept well out of reach. Instill in others who sometimes care for your loved one the importance of keeping a watchful eye. The benefits to you are obvious. It keeps injuries and stressful situations caused by accidents to a minimum.

JOURNAL KEEPING is sort of how this book came about. Throughout the years, I have jotted down my thoughts concerning experiences I have had as my husband's caregiver. You don't need any special talent to do this. It is similar to keeping a diary, only much less regimented. You don't have to write on a daily basis. Just pick up your pen whenever the spirit moves you.

There are personal feelings I wouldn't care to share with anyone else. Still, writing them out on paper is very therapeutic. It gets feelings out in the open, where you can see and deal with them. It lightens the load. If you want to keep what you've written from other people's eyes, one match will do the trick. Journal keeping is a very helpful aide to the caregiver. Try it—you'll like it.

JOYFUL COUNTENANCE may or may not describe your face, but don't forget to wear a smile in your daily struggles with the dependent. I know that when things get rough it is hard to look joyful, even if smiling does use fewer muscles. But remember, the show must go on, and a joyful countenance goes a long way in helping to get you both through a grin and bear it kind of day.

JUDGMENT, good judgment that is, is a wonderful quality to possess. It can certainly save us a heap of trouble, especially when we are teenagers. Usually though, it seems to be a little under-developed during those years. Hopefully, as we mature, our judgment capabilities improve.

As a caregiver, you will encounter a lot of situations that require good judgment. Don't expect to be one hundred percent in this department. When you are stressed out or tired, you won't always make the right decision for the moment. You can count on that. I find I do better if I can postpone making decisions at such times. Sleep on them, so to speak. If it is something major that needs deciding, I always seek advice from at least one person, or preferably two, whose judgment I trust. This way, if things don't work out as planned, we can share the blame. Learn from your mistakes and don't allow them too much fretting time.

JUMPING ROPE is good exercise and can be done indoors when the weather is wet. My daily schedule keeps me jumping, but that doesn't count.

I read recently that if you haven't got the time to walk or ride a bike, jumping rope, even a few minutes a day, is a very good way to get your exercise. At sixty-five, I doubt I'd last as long, or find it to be quite as much fun, as I did at age eight. But anything that can quickly get your tired blood circulating to your tired brain is worth a try. Now if I could just remember to buy a jump rope the next time I'm out shopping.

Janice Hucknall Snyder

K

KALEIDOSCOPES have always been fascinating to me. I love watching the changing colors. The stages of your life are like that. Changing patterns evolve as you are aging and experiencing life. Some patterns are bright and cheery, others dark and depressing, but still they are ever changing. If life seems gloomy now, wait. Just as the kaleidoscope turns into beautiful new colors, so will your life turn into happy times again. Believe it and look forward. In the meantime, it would help to find things to be happy and thankful for during the dark and sad times. That's difficult, but not impossible.

It is so very tragic to read about teenage suicides. You know that a lot of what is bothering them at such a young age wouldn't seem worth losing their precious lives over a few years down the road.

KEYS are the most frequently misplaced and searched for items that people own, besides glasses. Keep several extra house and car keys in different places: your office, your purse, with a trusted family member (some are not, you know—trusted, that is) or with a close neighbor, but never under the flowerpot or doormat. Being locked out of one's car or home is a dreadful experience, especially if it is raining, which is usually the case. If your dependent is with you, it can mean double trouble.

KINDNESS is something you need to share with others. It always improves the quality of your life. Sure, it takes a little time to do thoughtful things, but when people are down and out, a kind gesture can be just the boost they need to help them up again. You can't put a price on the value of that. A thoughtful "thinking of you" note or funny card can do wonders. Just ask Hallmark. If acts of kindness make one feel good, then caregivers should feel wonderful most of the time.

KISSES, like hugs, are a wonderful form of affection, and you can't get or give too many. Kissing is a smacking good habit for you and your dependent to share. It reinforces how much you care about each other.

KITCHENS are the most wonderful room in a house; at least that is so in our home. It is where children and grandchildren check out the Toll House cookies they could smell from a mile away and where cards and games are played while nibbling on crackers, popcorn or cheese; it is where the two ovens and the microwave can all be going at the same time while fudge is boiling on the stove, causing a wonderful aroma to permeate the house. The kitchen is always a focal point at parties and the source of much pleasure in our lives. It is also the room with the most dangers to a person with Alzheimer's disease or Dementia. Care should be taken to never leave this type of dependent alone in the kitchen. Accidents resulting in fires or burns could easily occur. Tap water may be left running because the person can't remember how to turn the faucet off. My husband often turns the spout to the back wall, thinking he is turning the faucet off. The water spreads rapidly over the counter top and cascades to the floor like a lovely waterfall. Splash! Grab the mop! Drinks also get spilled. Surviving as a caregiver includes not slipping in the kitchen and breaking a leg.

KNOWING what to do in every instance is not possible. Things happen sometimes which are beyond your comprehension and control. Seek help immediately. Don't dilly-dally when sudden physical or mental incidents happen that have the potential for danger to you or your dependent. Nobody wants to say, "If only I had." Regrets are hard to live with. They affect the quality of the rest of your life.

KNOWLEDGE is gained through a wonderful, exciting adventure in learning. Knowledge exercises your grey matter, keeps your mind growing and challenges you to think. Even though caregivers are often confined with the dependent person, they still have access to books, educational TV, home courses and other people's knowledge. Learning something new each day is a good habit to get into. It's hard to be depressed when you are being stimulated.

Janice Hucknall Snyder

L

LABELS in clothing help a lot if your dependent stays in a daycare facility or nursing home. Items will still disappear, but labels help when there's a mix-up. You can order pre-printed nametags on the Internet in all different colors. They have iron on ones and sew on ones. It is definitely easier and cheaper.

LAUGHTER is essential for the survival of anyone. A good hearty laugh is great for relieving stress. When you are dealing with an illness, it can be hard to find anything to laugh about. Try to see the comedy in situations, even situations where everything goes wrong. Things will happen that are better to laugh at than cry about. Both are a release, but laughter is more fun. And it's okay to be silly once in a while. Let the child in you come out to play. Lighten up.

It is not improper to have laughter in a home with a catastrophic illness. On the contrary, it helps to maintain a more normal balance and keep the dreaded depression at bay. If you are at a loss to find something funny to laugh about, there is always an old I Love Lucy show on TV to lift your spirits, and don't forget the newspaper comics. Laugh every chance you get, and share funny happenings with others. I have good friends who send me great jokes via e-mail.

LAWYERS are a necessity of life and death. Even if you've never felt the need to hire a lawyer, the circumstances of a catastrophic illness make it essential to have one. If there are assets (home, savings and checking accounts, stocks, etc.), they should all be transferred into the caregiver's name if he/she is the spouse. A good lawyer is required to handle these transactions and will advise you on your rights. At the same time, you should draw up a new will for yourself. That way, all the assets are passed on to the person or persons who will take over as caregiver should you die first. It does happen. The lawyer should also keep a copy of your Living Will.

Finances are critical when there is a catastrophic illness; the expenses are catastrophic too. The point may be reached when you can no longer do the caring and, in fact, need care yourself. If medical expenses take all your available money, the catastrophe is indeed complete. It is important for you to plan ahead. See to it that there are no assets in the dependent's name prior to the need to have the patient placed in a nursing home on Medicaid. Hopefully, it won't come down to that in your circumstances. I know that if all our assets were in my husband's name, it would leave me penniless and homeless in a few short years—sad, but true. My mom always said, "God helps those who help themselves."

Remember, you have to make these important decisions now. They will affect the quality of the rest of your life. You can't afford to put this off until tomorrow. Find a good lawyer to help keep you, the caregiver, solvent. You deserve no less.

LEISURE, what is that? It's what you would enjoy if you had any time left over after the three Cs: caring, cleaning and cooking. Time out is possible though, with planning and backup help. You should make every effort to "manipulate" leisure time into your daily schedule if you want to survive. Without it, life becomes a drudgery. So put those three Cs to work in a different way. Cut down on the cleaning and do more caring for yourself by cooking up some relaxing fun.

LIMITS are something we all have. Recognize that you have them too. There are times when circumstances are such that you think you can't slow down, as exhausted as you may be. Well, think again. At that point, it's time to send out an SOS to family or friends and take a break. It's for your own good, as well as the dependent's and yes, your family and friends' too. When you get past your limit, you become run down and vulnerable to illness. We already know that when the caregiver gets ill, it's double trouble for everyone. So pacing yourself and knowing your limits is a considerate way to go and a healthy rule to follow.

LISTENING, instead of planning what you'll say next, is the polite thing to do. You might even learn something. Everybody talked at once in our family, and nobody listened. It was a contest as to who could get the next word in edgewise. Consequently, I've never been a good listener, but I'm working on that. I admire that attribute in others a lot.

It is important to listen carefully to what the doctors say about your loved one's condition and the treatments to be given. That goes without saying. What your dependent says and the tone of voice they use can be an indication of how they are feeling. Listening helps you to monitor needs and moods. Your alertness can prevent added complications.

LITTLE THINGS mean a lot. They can also be your undoing. When you live with someone you love, there is a lot of give and take. You let a lot of little things that bother you go, only they aren't really going bye-bye. They are building up inside. One day, the other person will do something (any little, insignificant thing will do), and you will blow your top. The party getting the flack will probably say something like, "What are you getting so upset about? You act like there's been a disaster. All I did was put the toilet paper on backwards."

Then and there, you've reached your limit. You can't take it any longer. You have a volcanic reaction. Great balls of fire leap from your mouth—and it is all over a roll of toilet paper, or so the poor soul on the receiving end thinks. For everyone's sake, keep the lines of communication open. Don't go to bed with little gripes growling around inside of you, or you will wake up in bad humor, aggravated by a new addition, ULCERS.

LIVING WILLS are thoughtful documents that prevent a lot of suffering for patients and the loved ones standing by. There comes a time when the quality of life is such that one should be allowed to let go, move on. When the tubes going in and out of them are all that is keeping a person alive, that is not living. It is cruel, to say nothing of the exorbitant costs of such procedures. Do you feel strongly about the need for a Living Will to prevent this from happening to you or your loved one? Take the necessary steps to protect you both immediately. Be sure to use the Living Will form that is required in your state of residence. Your lawyer and/or the hospital should have the forms available. See that copies are given to your family members, doctor, religious leader and lawyer, so that there can be no doubt of your personal intentions concerning this matter. Keep the original in your safe deposit box.

LOOKING AHEAD realistically is a difficult thing to do, because in a catastrophic illness, the road gets bumpier and bumpier as you go along. The progression of an incurable illness involves coping with difficult changes, dealing with pain, making adjustments in the routine as needed and hoping the next stage is a long way off. I try not to think about the negative side of our tomorrows. Looking ahead, to the down side of the illness, is just too depressing to deal with day in and day out.

However, there are many important things concerning the illness that you must look ahead for and that you can't put on hold. The financial and legal concerns, the Living Will, etc., are important for you to think about and act on now. They are discussed in greater detail in other areas of this book.

LOVING and being loved is what life is all about. Without love, we are nothing. Caregivers know that love is unconditional and accept that. Loving is entwined with things I do as a caregiver, and it makes doing them a whole lot easier. I've had people say to me, "How can you do all that? How can you stand it?" The only answer I'm able to give is, "I love him. He's my husband. How could I not do it?"

I'm sure there are caregivers out there who have, because of extenuating circumstances, been forced to care for very unlovable people. That must be the most difficult of situations, truly a cross to bear. They need and deserve lots of help with this type of burden. May God bless them with great fortitude and many helpers.

LOWS happen to the caregiver as well as the ill person. You are supposed to be strong, brave and resourceful. You are to be all things to another human being who is totally dependent upon you. Just like a seesaw, you have your ups and downs.

When I feel low, it's usually because of one of the following: I'm sick and tired of everything I'm having to do, my loved one is having a bad day, the taxes just went up again on our home, three things broke down in the house (it always happens in threes), I wasn't able to find time for swimming this week, or friends just stopped by to tell me they are off to Europe for three weeks. There are many reasons for "lows." I'm sure you've experienced your share as a caregiver. I'm sure you could add to my list.

When a low hits, I have to quickly take stock of all the blessings we've had and remind myself that things could always be worse. That helps me climb back up out of the pit. Next, I go out and buy myself something special. It could be a new blouse or an ice cream cone at my favorite place. Do whatever works for you, just as long as it gets you up and out of the blues as quickly as possible.

LUCK is winning the lottery, and how! That sure would help with money worries, but I'll settle for all the other good luck I can get, especially since bad luck usually comes in bunches. In a period of three weeks' time, the company my husband worked for went belly up, he was diagnosed with Parkinson's disease and, subsequently, he was hospitalized with a nervous breakdown. Three strikes: we were down, but not out. We've had bunches of good luck along the way too.

Survival of the Caregiver

Everyone who lives long enough gets a share of both kinds of luck. That's life. Make the most of your good luck. Try not to dwell on the bad, that's a downer. Downers are hard on your survival.

Janice Hucknall Snyder

M

MAINTENANCE of your body is a must. Just as your car requires regular attention in order to perform properly, so do you. Don't put off routine physical examinations and dental check-ups. Watch your consumption of the foods you love so much; you know, the ones that aren't good for your cholesterol, blood pressure and weight. Eat in moderation, and eat sensibly to avoid health problems that could then require you to be on a restricted, no fun diet.

Exercise keeps our body tuned up and trimmed down. It should be done on a regular basis, not in spurts. Never overtax your body by doing doubles after you missed a day. Use your common sense. When I see an older person jogging in ninety-five-degree weather looking totally exhausted, I say to myself, "There goes a heart attack waiting to happen."

Maintenance on the dwelling you share with your dependent is another expensive, time-consuming task. Things tend to break down in bunches. Keep ahead of the game with preventive maintenance wherever possible. In our old house, built in 1917, there's always something that needs hammering or painting. This is where it is great to have strong, handy and willing sons and sons-in-law. Mine are a tremendous help in the repair department. God bless them all.

MAKEOVERS are uplifting to your face and your spirits. Have you ever had one? It is really a fun thing to do. I was feeling in a rut (caregivers do get in them) when I noticed an ad in the newspaper. It said a cosmetologist would be at a certain department store the following week, he would be doing makeovers for FREE, and to call and make an appointment. I felt rather ridiculous, but needing a change of any sort and knowing that traveling around the world was out, I quickly dialed the number before I could change my mind. I figured that at sixty-five, I really was overdue for a new face. Surprisingly enough, I even liked the new look. It was just what the doctor ordered. It gave me a real lift, while deflating my pocketbook. The makeover was free, as advertised, but the cosmetics I bought to keep my new look going were not. My big splurge was still well worth it, mentally and physically. Look good, feel good. . . look bad, feel bad. A makeover does the trick. Go for it.

MASSAGES make your body feel happy all over, or so they say. I've never had a real one, where you go to a massage parlor, take off all your clothes and somebody kneads your body for an hour. It sounds wonderful though and comes highly recommended. I have put that on my "Things I Want to Do" list. Then there's the Jacuzzi hot tub. I've never had one of those either, but I have enjoyed soaking in one at a spa.

On the practical side, there's the "good pal" kind of massage. That's where you tell whoever is closest, "Hey, would you please just rub my neck and back a little, right there?" Then you ooh and aah a lot while he/she is doing the rubbing to keep them from stopping. It helps if you return the favor; that way you might have a massage buddy for life. It is another aide to surviving as a caregiver.

The ill person you're caring for needs daily massages to keep blood circulating and muscles toned up, especially if bed-ridden.

MASTURBATION is a tension getter. This is a closed subject to you if your mind has been programmed to think negatively about it, but self-gratification can be an excellent way of relieving tension. The benefit is invaluable to someone dealing with stressful situations on a daily basis. In turn, when you are more relaxed, you send good signals to the person you are caring for. See more on this subject under "INTERCOURSE."

MEDICAID is the program you turn to as a last resort. In dealing with a catastrophic illness, you never know what the situation will be in one or two years. How will your patient be physically and financially? How will you be? That is why I emphasize the need to make sure that all of the patient's assets are legally handled well ahead of time. It ensures his/her eligibility for Medicaid, yet doesn't leave you, the caregiver, destitute.

To emphasis the importance of this, I would like to tell you of a case I heard about recently. A friend's aunt was placed into a nursing home under Medicaid. It is the government's policy to cash in all of the assets of anyone entering a nursing home on Medicaid. This lady had prepaid all of her funeral arrangements. Medicaid subsequently confiscated and cashed in the prepaid funeral plan, along with all of her other assets. They don't overlook anything. Some people actually divorce their partners so that Medicaid will not confiscate 50% of their total assets. This seems drastic, but when the caregiver is over sixty-five, with meager assets left, and unable to work, desperation sets in quickly. It is a sad state of affairs, to say the least.

MEDICARE is something you get when you turn an age you don't want to be. It sure does help with the insurance costs though.

I have worked in a doctor's office for many years, and I have spent a lot of time trying to help people understand what it means when a doctor "Accepts Assignment." Patients have the misconception (or maybe they have wishful thinking) that when the doctor accepts what Medicare allows for a procedure, the patient doesn't have to pay anything. Wrong. The patient still has to pay 20% of the approved amount. For example: if the charge is $100.00 and Medicare approves $80.00, the doctor has to write off the difference of $20.00. Of the $80.00 approved amount, Medicare pays 80%, which is $64.00. The patient's responsibility is 20%, which is $16.00. If the patient has a supplemental second insurance, it will pick up and pay the $16.00 balance. But remember, some insurance policies have deductibles to be met first. Be sure you know how much your deductibles are. I had a patient who kept insisting his secondary insurance should pay. It was his understanding that everything Medicare didn't pay, his other insurance would. In checking with his secondary insurance company, we found out that the deductible in his insurance contract was $1,500.00. It would take a long time before 20% of his medical expenses exceeded that amount. Always check your contracts carefully. Did you know that federal law requires physicians to collect the deductible and 20% co-payment from their patients? Failure to do so is illegal. Patients shouldn't ask or expect their doctors to accommodate them with an additional write off. Medicare has cut back the approved amounts paid to many doctors drastically already.

MEDICATIONS are exorbitant money. Just dealing with that expense is worrisome enough. My husband's medications cost over $700.00 a month. Fortunately, my supplemental insurance pays 75% of some prescriptions and 50% of others. However, it still costs me approximately $200.00 per month, plus $190.00 for the supplemental insurance coverage.

A friend of mine was shocked recently when she picked up a prescription for her husband at the drug store; it was fifty pills to be taken over a period of two weeks. The cost was $1,489.00. Fortunately, her insurance covers all but $10.00 on any prescription. What do people do that don't have that kind of insurance? Go without? Die? (See "Prescriptions" for further information.)

Aside from the expense factor, medications are a very essential and important part of caring for an ailing person. Just keeping up with the schedule is a job. My husband takes a variety of pills, seven times a day. If I get busy and forget to give him his medications for half an hour, his whole system slows to the point that he can't walk. I purchased a timer that can be set for three different times at once. It is a good reminder, if I'm near enough to hear it when it goes off. A wristwatch with an alarm that beeps would solve that problem, but I'd probably forget to set it.

Dispensing the pills to the patient can be still another problem. My husband gets very stubborn at times and refuses to take his medication, even though his mobility depends on it. He doesn't understand; he just knows he's tired of taking all those awful pills. As awful as they are, he will pretend to take them, hold them in his mouth for half an hour and then spit the now liquid pills out. Yuk! Exasperating, to say the least. If you have problems with your dependent taking medications, try breaking or crushing the pills and mixing them with jelly or applesauce. Do not crush time-released pills. Watch carefully to see that the pills get swallowed. Ask the patient to open his/her mouth if you aren't sure they went down. I've discovered many pills stuck on the tongue.

There are all kinds of containers you can buy to keep pills in proper order. Find the type that suits your needs best, such as daily or weekly setups. Containers help you keep track and save you from having to unscrew several different bottles at pill time.

The latest "good" news on TV is that you can't trust your druggist either. Now we are supposed to count the pills because some druggists purposely short-change us. This is sad, but true, and it is time consuming to do.

Always read directions carefully for drugs; be sure to check the side effects. Doctors are not perfect, and certain drugs can have serious side effects when a patient has other conditions. You know better than anyone what conditions your dependent has. Beware! No matter how great a "wonder" drug is, there are always some people who cannot tolerate it or who are allergic to it. There could be serious adverse reactions, even to the point of death. In line with this, everyone should always carry a list of all the drugs they are taking in their wallets. People are very lax about this. From my experience working for an Ophthalmologist, I would say 65% of our patients can't remember what drugs they are taking and fail to bring in a list. "I didn't think I would need one. I'm just having my eyes checked" is the usual comment. These are people with heart conditions, high blood pressure, diabetes, glaucoma, asthma, rheumatoid arthritis, etc. They are all taking lots of medications. Certain medications cannot be taken with other medications.

How is a doctor to know if you don't bring the information with you? He must take time to call your other physicians or wait for you bring in a list before he can prescribe what you need.

Even more important, God forbid, what if you and your loved one are in an accident and both unconscious? The medics will check your wallet. Will they find a card there saying how much insulin you need, that you have an implant in your right eye, that you are wearing contact lenses? Remember to update this list every time you change medications and dosages.

Some dos on medications: do flush down the toilet any drugs you are told to discontinue or that are outdated, do check with your doctor on the timing for taking the prescription (before, with or after meals), do avoid foods if indicated, as with some medications and do keep medications out of the reach of children and people with dementia and depression.

MEMORIES are a source of renewal and play a vital roll in the caregiver's life. Are things not going well? Are you feeling blue? Draw on the memories of special times in your life. They can give you just the boost you need. Get out the old family photo albums. They are fun to look through and help jar your memories of the good times.

Hopefully you've stored up lots of happy memories along the way by living an active life so there will be no regrets when your activities are drastically curtailed.

It is equally important to let go of the bad memories of failures and mistakes; they are the stuff that depressions are made of. You don't have the time or energy for depression.

MIRACLES are gifts beyond our comprehension from a higher power. When I taught Sunday school, I had no trouble explaining what a miracle looked like. I merely pulled a snapshot out of my wallet and showed it to the class. It was a picture of our youngest daughter, Susie, when she weighed 1 lb. 5 oz. The nurse's hands, hovering over her tiny body, looked large by comparison. She was three whole months premature. The kids in my class all knew Susie, so there was no need for words. They could see she was a normal, happy, healthy child. Susie is now a nurse in the Neo-Natal Intensive Care Unit at a hospital, taking care of tiny babies just like her. But that is the second part of my miracle story. The first miracle was two months before Susie was born. Our one-year-old son, Gary, had developed a rare allergic reaction to a viral infection. This syndrome had a very low survival rate. Usually, if the child did survive, they suffered brain damage and blindness. Gary made a complete recovery—nothing less than a miracle in my mind. That's two miracles in three months. When I'm down and out, remembering all those miracles gets me up fast. Do I believe in miracles? You bet I do! And yes, prayers are answered. So never stop hoping and praying for miracles; they can become realities.

MOON. If it's full, look out. I never put too much store in the power of the moon. That was Hollywood stuff, with werewolves and other monsters creeping through fog enshrouded forests. Then a nurse working on the Alzheimer's floor of a nursing home straightened me out. She said that when the moon was full, there was always a great deal of unrest in the nursing home and many more problems in dealing with the patients there. Observing my husband the next full moon, I realized that she was right. He was much more confused, and tended to get angry and upset a lot more easily. (There is definitely power in the gravitational pull of the moon; just look how it controls the tides in the ocean.)

I dread the approach of the full moon. Keeping calm, cool and collected is a challenge during those four or five days. After one frightening session, I realized I needed more than patience to deal with the problem. My husband's doctor prescribed a mild tranquilizer for three days before the full moon and two days after. My calendar is well marked. This doesn't totally eliminate outbursts, but it helps with the more aggressive ones. Fortunately, your loved one will become more lovable shortly thereafter. Be alert to mood swings; it could keep you from having to duck an arm swing.

MURPHY'S LAW, also known as "Shit Happens," is an experience we have all had at least a dozen times in our lives. If anything can go wrong, it no doubt will, so count on it. Think of it as a challenge, never a defeat, and you will survive.

MUSIC is not only food for the soul; it warms the heart and fills us with contentment. It makes me want to sing, clap my hands and dance. When I put on an "Oldies" tape, I'm hit with nostalgia. Listening to Bing Crosby and Grace Kelly singing "True Love," transports me back to when I got married. We chose that oldie for our first dance, and we danced cheek to cheek. Remembering better times, when my husband was whole, always gives me a lift. It is good to connect with happy memories of the loved one we're caring for. The past gives meaning to the present. It keeps what two people mean to each other alive, even when one is no longer sure who the other is anymore. So have music playing from dawn to dusk. Keep those happy memories alive and your spirits soaring.

Janice Hucknall Snyder

N

NEEDS are something we all have, not just the disabled, who obviously have many. I think it is very important for the disabled person to recognize that the caregiver has needs too. The only way that can happen is through complete honesty between the two of you.

I spare my husband the problems I have to deal with daily. But I do want him to know that I need to be hugged a lot, I need his support and understanding when I'm tired, and at times, I even need to have a "time out" from caring for him.

Keep the lines of communication open. Discuss each other's needs as long as it is possible. It will be beneficial to both of you.

NEGATIVE THINKING should be avoided as much as possible. This is easier said than done when you are a caregiver. A person with a catastrophic illness is going to have degrees of depression. Where there is depression, negative thinking is close behind. It can be catching. Recognize when your own negative thoughts are taking over and cut them short. Negative thinking is insidious and can creep up on you before you know it. Stay alert. Counteract such thoughts with positive ones. Get involved in an activity that is stimulating, quick.

NEGLECT of your own needs happens. Quite naturally, the dependent's needs come first. That automatically makes the caregiver's needs second, third or even fourth if there are other family members living with you.

Getting your own personal priorities straight requires some soul-searching. Some things will have to be neglected. You have to decide which things are the most important to you. Put the rest of your interests at the bottom of the list, to be retrieved if and when there is time. People who believe cleanliness is next to Godliness will put keeping the house in perfect order at the top of the list. People who are artistic may think that should be last on the list. To each his own! It doesn't matter how you arrange your list. There is no right or wrong way. Just make sure the things you like to do the most are at the top of the list and get done. Don't neglect yourself, or you will be a very unhappy, barely surviving caregiver.

NEIGHBORS, God bless them, every one. We have been very fortunate in that we have lived in the same house for thirty-seven years. Most of our neighbors have been around a long time too. We have "5th Street" parties, which grow and change each year, plus a Kentucky Derby Party with our neighbors. These warm, caring folks are an important part of our lives, especially now that we don't go out as much. They know the circumstances of my husband's illness and respond to him appropriately. Our neighbors could and would come to my aid if need be. There is comfort in knowing that. Hopefully you live in a warm and friendly neighborhood like mine. Neighbors can play a meaningful part in the caregiver's life. One or two neighbors should be made aware of the basic routine and drugs given. It doesn't hurt to have extra back-ups.

NERVOUSNESS is something you experience when you are taking an important exam, giving a speech, going for your first job interview, getting married or heading for the hospital to have your first baby.

There is also nervousness caused by the constant stress and strain of caring for a failing loved one. There will be times when the whole scenario makes you want to scream. That would probably be the best thing you could do for yourself at that moment.

When I get too uptight, and my nervous energy abounds, I do something physical to release the tension, even if it's simply taking slow, deep breaths or stretching.

I know someone whose husband had a Grand Mall Seizure. It has affected his thinking ever since. Now there are times when he asks the same question six or seven times. She will answer the question, and a few minutes later he will ask it again. This is nerve-wracking to say the least.

Nerves affect your whole body, so they should be taken seriously. I'm talking survival here. When your nervous system short circuits, it is called a nervous breakdown. When that happens, you are the one needing a caregiver. So don't ignore warning signals: inability to sleep, sleeping too much, lack of appetite, no energy, too much energy, lack of interest in your personal appearance or crying, to name a few. Take a break before you break.

NEUTRAL, in a car, is when it's just idling; it isn't going anywhere. A caregiver doesn't have the time to be in neutral very often, there is always so much to do. But it is a good idea to put on your brakes and slow down to neutral for at least thirty minutes a day. That is, if you want to get the greatest mileage out of your body.

Janice Hucknall Snyder

NO doesn't always mean no when your patient has Alzheimer's or another form of Dementia. So look out! When your question is answered with a no, it could mean yes. "Do you need to go to the bathroom?" Answer, "no." Don't you believe it. Then again, the answer could be "yes," but after getting the dependent into the bathroom and unbuckling their pants, there's no need. The word frustrating describes these kinds of experiences. The solution would be to not ask questions, but it's the natural thing to do when checking on your dependent's needs. Think of this part of your care giving as a challenging guessing game. Call it, "Out-guessing the Patient and Surviving." Otherwise, you might not.

NOISE is one of the biggest pollutants in the world today. It pollutes our minds. It resounds from TVs, radios, CDs and DVDs played at full volume. The remote control was a spectacular invention. I get great satisfaction from muting the commercials that come blasting on twenty decibels louder.

Our three teenage grandsons stayed with us recently for a week. That was an experience in noise. They are all experts at getting each other in trouble with their parents, and when one starts something, the rest finish it. This scene is always "enriched" with loud screaming and vying to get one person's side of the story heard above the others. My kingdom for a remote control that would tune them out as quickly as the TV! Now that's a necessity that needs inventing, but don't misunderstand me. I love my grandchildren.

An excess of noise can be very stressful for you and your loved one. Naturally, a peaceful atmosphere is more restful and easier on your nerves. If this means limiting visitors, especially noisy ones, don't hesitate to let your feelings be known.

NUISANCE is a word caregivers have no trouble relating to. Lots of things happen when you are caring for an ill person that are a nuisance. I call them "grin and bear it" situations.

My husband misplaces his glasses regularly. I remember one time, I searched the house from top to bottom. When our grandson stopped by, he joined the hunt. His incentive was the dollar bill I dangled in front of his face. He searched with great furor, to no avail. Two days later, I spotted the glasses outside on the deck. The good news was that no one had stepped on them. Using my hindsight, I got a strap to put on the glasses. Hopefully, that will solve the problem. Searching for things is such an aggravation. It is a waste of valuable time, which would be better spent on your favorite hobby.

Nuisances take a lot out of you and try your patience. Eliminate the cause of an annoyance at the first opportunity, if not sooner.

NURSING HOME care for the dependent may eventually become the only means of your survival. The ill person's condition may deteriorate and require specialized care. Your loved one's degree of agitation might become severe, uncontrollable and dangerous to your wellbeing. You may develop health problems. A nursing home, at such times, is not only a viable consideration: it's a responsible, affirmative decision.

Check out every nursing home facility in your area. Take someone along with you to help; four eyes and ears are better than two. Take along a list of prepared questions about the qualifications and routines of the facility. Get a tour of every area, including the kitchen. Odors are hard to control in a nursing facility, but some do a far better job of controlling them than others. The less odor, the more likely it is that patients are regularly changed and sanitation procedures are strictly adhered to. If the nursing home you believe to be the best is farther away than you'd like, drive the extra distance. Your peace of mind is worth it.

The ideal alternative to a nursing home is having someone qualified come in and take charge of your loved one. This is only possible for those who are very secure financially. Otherwise, start looking into nursing home care before there is a real need. That way, when the time is at hand, you will know what you want to do. Some nursing homes, especially the nicest ones, have waiting lists. If you have put your loved one's name on the list early, the wait to get admitted will be lessened.

Even if your loved one is already on disability insurance and/or Medicare, you still need to apply for Medicaid to cover this tremendous expense. Assets should be transferred out of the disabled person's name before applying for this aid. This is a state run program, so check requirements for when assets should be transferred from the disabled person's name and also check for how much the disabled can own in the way of assets. If your loved one doesn't meet these criteria, the cost will be much higher for nursing home care. (See MEDICAID for further information.) For the average, middle class family, these costs are catastrophic. The caregiver would be destitute within a few years, or less. Surviving wouldn't be much fun then.

If you haven't already planned ahead, act now to get the dependent's affairs in order so he/she will be qualified. If I am being somewhat repetitious on this subject, it is because it is so critical to the survival of the caregiver.

NUTRITION is an essential part of the caregiver's survival. Well-balanced meals, fresh fruit, vegetables and roughage in the diet keep you healthy and energetic.

A proper diet for the dependent is also important. Food for patients who have difficulty chewing or swallowing should be cut in small pieces or blended. Add Ensure as a dietary supplement if the patient is losing weight. Both of you should take vitamins daily to cover all the bases.

Janice Hucknall Snyder

O

OBLIGATIONS require fulfillment. They are things you are bound to follow through on because of a promise made, rules of etiquette, your relationship, favors owed, etc.

When I feel obligated to do something, it somehow loses its appeal. It's like I'd rather not, but for whatever reason, I'd better get it done. I don't like writing thank you notes, fixing lunch for the boss at the office, or getting all dressed up in the middle of the week.

If you became a caregiver because you felt obligated to do so, that could make surviving more difficult. When resentfulness creeps into your thinking, it makes care giving all the more tedious. Care giving is challenging enough when it is done out of love.

OBSTACLES in caring for your loved one are always just around the corner. When they come in bunches, duck! Take a breather and cool it. Regroup!

Example: The obstacle was constipation. I had given my husband a laxative in a last ditch effort to avoid having to give a Fleet's Enema (one of my very least favorite things to do). The timing was somehow off. There were false alarms at 1 a.m., 3:30 a.m. and 6 a.m. Then it was time to rise and shine for work. Two more "attempts" made getting to work on time impossible. Dropping my husband off at the day center, I breathed a sigh of relief. The problem was in their hands now. With a heavy foot on the gas pedal and a yawn, I headed for the office. After work, I was dragging, but glad everything would have come out okay by now. Wrong: the best was yet to come, three rounds later. Needless to say, the rest of that laxative was trashed. Even a Fleet's enema is easier than that. Subsequently, my husband's doctor gave me a prescription for a liquid laxative that works just right.

Obstacles are difficult at best when having to care for someone. If at all possible, find a way to get around them rather than deal with them. Foresight is better than hindsight, but experience is usually the best teacher.

ONE DAY AT A TIME is all a caregiver can handle when things are in a critical stage for the dependent. You can't be like Scarlet O'Hara and say, "I'll think about that tomorrow, after all, tomorrow is another day."

You have to deal with situations as they happen. If the problem seems gigantic, tell yourself, "Today is all I have to be concerned with, right now." Concentrate all your energies on getting through the present crisis or situation. Having to deal with anything else would be too much. Controlling stress is vital to keeping a clear head and to your survival.

OPEN-MINDEDNESS is a beneficial attribute for the caregiver. It is so easy to get set in our way of thinking.

When I am doing all the caring and someone suggests a way I could do something better, I am not always receptive. Sometimes I am even resentful. When I'm tired or in a bad mood, I might interpret it as an indication that the person thinks I'm not doing a good job. I could even be upset that I didn't think of it first.

People have different life experiences to draw from. When you keep an open mind, you are able to concede that other people's ideas could benefit the patient and/or ease your work. Then you are able to consider and accept constructive criticism graciously. People do mean well. My mom always said, "I'm only telling you for your own good." Once in a while I believed her, because she was right.

OPHTHALMOLOGISTS are surgeons skilled in dealing with every condition of the eye. Don't take chances with such a precious thing as sight. For complete eye care, never depend on an Optician or Optometrist. Only the Ophthalmologist is a licensed doctor who can perform surgery on the eye. People with Diabetes can get Diabetic Retinopathy and a subsequent loss of vision. High Blood Pressure can affect the eyes. Pressure in the eyes should be checked regularly to prevent blindness from Glaucoma. Visual Fields can detect a loss of peripheral vision from Glaucoma, and the extent of visual loss from strokes, tumors or changes in the optic nerve. There are many eye conditions that only an Ophthalmologist would have the expertise to detect and treat properly in time.

The doctor I work for is an Ophthalmologist. He didn't tell me to say all this. I am speaking from the heart-breaking experience of seeing people lose their vision because they waited too long to see an Ophthalmologist. Please do get regular eye check-ups for your dependent and yourself. Total darkness is not a pretty sight.

OPTIMISM is an upper. If you don't have an optimistic attitude when you are a caregiver, pessimism takes over. Pessimism is a downer. Before you know it, everything becomes negative. From there, it's a short hop, skip and jump into that disheartening word, depression. Now I don't need to tell you that a depressed person taking care of a depressed person equals an impossibility. So, whatever it takes to keep you optimistic about your lot in life, do it. See "ATTITUDE" under "A." People quickly get tired of listening to negative people. Don't dwell on all the problems you have to deal with, or pretty soon, nobody will be around to listen.

ORGANIZATION saves time. If you are a slob, you are lost, and so are your things. "Once a slob, always a slob?" I hope not, because if you can't change this way of life, life will be much more difficult for you as a caregiver. One of the most important things in your life now is time. Time spent looking for misplaced things is time taken away from you. "A place for everything and everything in its place" is a good way to keep organized and will save you hours of looking. The secret to making all of this work is to put everything you use back where it belongs as soon as you are finished using it. Then it will be there the next time you need it.

My mother was the most unorganized person in the world. Maybe that's why I'm the opposite. If there was an unexpected knock at the door, all of us kids were trained to grab things and throw them in the closet. Mom spent hours looking for things. She drove us all nuts by talking about the lost object the whole time she was looking for it. It went something like this; "I know I put it somewhere in here. Have you seen it, Janice? Did you take it? Someone must have moved it. What could have happened to it? Oh dear, isn't this just terrible, wherever could it be? I'm lost without it." On and on it went until she would finally find it, right where she had left it, much to everyone's relief. I've been organized ever since.

OUTINGS may be difficult to manage, but it is important to get you both out of the house as much as possible, even if you just go for a drive around the neighborhood.

I can remember the good 'ole days when the highlight of the week was when Daddy piled the whole family in the Ford. Off we'd go for a Sunday drive. Try to get kids away from TV or video games long enough to do that today. As if you could get them to do such a boring thing, unless you were headed for a shopping mall.

If your dependent has serious mobility problems, there are various kinds of mechanical aides to facilitate movement. One lady comes to our office in a motorized wheelchair. She then transfers herself to a harness lift contraption that raises her from the wheel chair to the examination chair with ease. It is a large piece of equipment, but it folds and separates into manageable parts. Her daughter drives a large van with a special lift on the side. It raises the wheel chair up and into the van and provides adequate space for the harness lift. The harness lift is something that they rent from a Medical Supply Company. Medicare covers most of the expense. This lady is totally paralyzed. Without these aides, her daughter would never be able to handle her transportation needs, even in the house. Many people don't realize that there is excellent equipment available to aid with mobility problems.

When my dependent has an appointment with the doctor, dentist, etc., it helps to plan well in advance. When being on time is a factor, I get pretty harried if something happens to delay our departure. That can be hard on the blood pressure. I try to get everything ready ahead of time. I know full well that some unforeseen situation will no doubt occur to slow the process and delay our departure. I do my best when I figure it all out backwards, starting with the time I have to arrive at the doctor's office: say, 10 a.m. I need half an hour to get there, so I'll leave at 9:30, which means breakfast will be ready at 8:30 a.m., so I'll start making it at 8:10 a.m. It takes one hour to dress the two of us, so dressing my husband begins at 7:10. This means I need to rise and shine at 7 a.m. to give myself an extra ten-minute leeway. Hopefully, the night before, I made a list of questions for the doctor, updated the list of medications to give the doctor, put enough pills in the pillbox to cover Richard's needs while we are away from the house and set out a container of water to have in the car for taking pills. There is less stress on me the day of the outing if everything is handled ahead of time. Again, controlling stress is the name of the game.

OVERWHELMED is a feeling the caregiver is very familiar with. The reality, the responsibility, the devastation to your loved one, the daily struggles, the worry, and the financial burden can at times close in on you in an overwhelming way. At such times, I call on a higher power to renew my faith and confidence. I shut the door on all my worries and remind myself, once again, that today is all I have to handle for now. This is much less intimidating. This is manageable.

P

PATIENCE OF A SAINT is an expression I often heard my mother use. "Raising you four kids takes the patience of a saint," she would say in her frustration.

I learned patience from a schoolteacher, but not in the classroom; it was on a tennis court. She challenged me every three weeks for my position on the tennis ladder. We would go as many as twenty-four games to decide one set. I was younger and taller, but she was smarter and lobbed over me every time I rushed the net to put the ball away. It was the most frustrating experience. I had to play her game and keep my patience in order to win the matches. They were long and grueling in ninety-five degree heat. Nothing tested my patience like that, until I became a caregiver.

I don't really have the patience of a saint. I'm far from it. I do try very hard to not lose my cool when my husband does something upsetting that causes me extra work though. Nevertheless, it happens, and me shouting, "Why did you do that?" is very upsetting to him. It is also a stupid question. People with Dementia or Alzheimer's are like little children. In their confusion, they don't realize that what they are doing may be a problem for someone else.

Janice Hucknall Snyder

They don't even know why they are being yelled at. I have noticed that when I start yelling at him in anger, I'm usually overtired, proving the importance of getting sufficient rest. I don't feel good about losing my patience, but I realize there will be times when I run out of it. You will, too.

Caregivers are entitled to a good yell once in a while. It clears the air and releases pent up feelings of frustration.

PEACE OF MIND is a wonderful attainment. In our church, we pray God will grant us peace, which passes all understanding. Inner peace gives one serenity, strength and courage—all needs of the caregiver. Pray for it daily. Try to avoid interactions that cause turmoil and upset. That's easier said than done.

PEOPLE, in general, are very understanding and nice when they realize someone is disabled. Then there are others who can't help but stare. They make you feel uncomfortable and upset, as well as your loved one. That is not a good feeling. Humans are a naturally curious lot. When there is an automobile accident on the road, there are always a lot of "rubberneckers" making the slow down even worse.

Working in a Doctor's office, I attend to a lot of disabled and disfigured people. It is important to be perceptive in handling such persons, to make them feel at ease. Deep down inside, they are beautiful, brave souls, who are very deserving of everyone's respect. If you didn't realize that before you were a caregiver, you certainly do now.

PETS can be such fun and such trouble. When the children were young, we always had a dog and/or outside cat. I've come very close, many times, to getting a dog for my husband, because a pet is good therapy for a disabled and depressed person. Besides that, I love Dachshunds and

English Springer Spaniels. I was close to getting a Spaniel one time. The puppies had just been born. I was going to pick one out of the litter that evening. Then I made one of those lists where you write down all the reasons why you should get a dog and all the reasons why you shouldn't get a dog. The list with, "messes to clean up, stains on the rug, fleas, chewed furniture, hair everywhere, dog left alone all day, and walking day and night, rain or shine," won out. But if I were able to stay home all day, I think I would be inclined to take on the extra work, because pets, for a disabled person, can be such a wonderful, enjoyable distraction. Parakeets or fish are less work, but it's pretty hard to hug a bird or fish.

PLAN your work and work your plan. At my graduation from grammar school, one of the speakers used that phrase for the theme of his talk to the class. That was fifty-three years ago. He did a good job of making his point with me, didn't he? I can't remember anything else about the speaker, but I'm sure he would be pleased if he knew how much those words influenced my life. I have followed that rule ever since. I do plan my activities and goals, and I do work until I achieve them. It's a good way to get things done. If I have chores and fun activities planned, I won't let myself do the fun things until the chores are done and out of the way. It's amazing how fast I can go when there's a fun goal.

Planning your work and working your plan is even more meaningful when you are a caregiver. This system will help you to keep on top of daily needs and, more important, provide you with time for a variety of diversions.

PLASTIC is a wonder. I bless the day that it was discovered, even though I know it is an environmental hazard to be dealt with. I appease my conscious by recycling.

Janice Hucknall Snyder

There are so many ways that plastic benefits the caregiver: plastic sheets to save the mattress, plastic diapers to control waste products, plastic non-breakable cups with lids, plastic bags to contain garbage, etc. I guess we caregivers could manage without it if we had to, but I'd sure hate to have to try. I always buy plastic products in the super large, economy size. I shop at the discount stores with the lowest prices on these types of products. Some wholesale stores don't accept coupons, but at the stores that do, those savings add up.

POSITIVE THINKING is recognized as an invaluable attitude to possess. It strengthens one's views concerning all things one must deal with. This, in turn, makes positive thinking easier to attain. Google Amazon; there are many books out there that can help. My favorite is the classic: The Power of Positive Thinking by Dr. Norman. It is good reading for the caregiver.

POWER OF ATTORNEY is an important document for you to have when dealing with the legal affairs of your dependent. Time is of the essence if your dependent is progressing with Alzheimer's or Dementia. This transference of authority to you, the agent, is only possible while the person giving the power can do so with a sound mind and with full awareness of what he/she is doing. Do not procrastinate on this important issue. The document should be notarized and kept with other important papers in a safe deposit box. Keep a copy at home for easy access when proof is needed.

PRAYER helps to get you through the bad times when you feel totally unable to deal with care giving. There are times when the condition of my husband is such that praying is the only thing I know to do to help us both. Believe in the power of prayer. When my husband isn't able to communicate well, I feel very alone. It's good to know that I have an understanding listener "upstairs," keeping a line open for me. God gives me an extra boost of inner-strength when I need it the most. I call on Him a lot. Amen.

PREPARATIONS are made when a couple is about to have a child; they prepare for the birth. The child prepares for being an adult by going to school; he/she prepares for life. Each day, you prepare for the day; you prepare for the activities that need to be done. Ultimately, caregivers must also prepare for the possibility that their loved one will pass on. For that, you must prepare legally, but you can never be totally prepared in your heart. That is the very hardest part of being a caregiver.

PRESCRIPTIONS don't cost the same at every drug store. Shop around. If you've used a conveniently located druggist for years, you tend to continue doing so when you are suddenly confronted with paying for several expensive drugs. Like your doctor, you trust him and have faith in his ability to fill your prescriptions properly. You even have him diagnose your little ailments, so shopping around for lower prices doesn't seem necessary. After all, there couldn't be that much difference in the costs, could there? Unfortunately, the answer is yes. I got a card in the mail from AARP saying that if I would send them the names, strengths and amounts of each of the drugs my dependent used, they would send me a quote of what the drugs would cost through AARP. Just out of curiosity, I filled out the card and sent it in. What a shock I got when the quote came back. The difference in price per year for two drugs was $750.00. Rather significant, don't you think? Needless to say, I pick up the phone once a month now and call an 800 number to order my husband's drugs through AARP.

Janice Hucknall Snyder

They send two copies of the bill: one for my records and one to file with the insurance claim. The insurance company pays them directly. It's as simple as that.

Unless your insurance pays all but $10.00 on each of your prescriptions, it would pay you to shop around and get quotes from several drug stores. If you are fifty-five or older, join AARP and take advantage of their savings. If you receive Medicare, you can be in their prescription plan or you can join other companies for a big savings on prescriptions. One of those is Humana. Check them all out.

PREVENTION, remember the saying? "An ounce of prevention is worth a pound of cure." That says it all. Taking steps to prevent problems or complications from happening saves you big worries and expenses down the road. Just as with a car, preventive maintenance with the body keeps you running smoothly. Proper sleep, diet, vitamins, check-ups, recreation, attitude, etc., can make a difference in caregivers and dependents alike.

PRIORITIES in your life have to focus on the person you are caring for—his/her comfort and well-being. But a close second would be the well-being of you, yourself, for obvious reasons. All the rest of your needs, even money, have less of a priority. Although, let it be said, I would never underestimate the need for money when dealing with a catastrophic illness. I guess money would be a close third on the priority list. Keeping your priorities straight isn't difficult when you are a caregiver; these three being the nucleus. Handle all others when you can.

PROBLEMS are something we could all do without, but they happen anyway. Don't be like an ostrich with its head in the sand, because problems don't usually go away by themselves. Quite the opposite, they can snowball. Deal with situations directly; it saves a lot of trouble and worry in the long run.

PSYCHIATRISTS . . . there are psychiatrists, and then there are psychiatrists. Just as in any profession, some are better than others. There is also the important element of finding a doctor that the ill person can relate to and feel comfortable with. A doctor might be excellent and well recommended to you, but if there is no charisma between two people, nothing else will work. Keep looking.

Psychiatrists mainly prescribe medications to relieve the systems of stress, anxiety and stages of depression. Their function is to give the right dosages of the right medications so that the patient's systems (mental and physical) run like a Mercedes instead of a Jalopy. Then the patient can deal with all the things that are happening in his/her life that got him/her in that condition in the first place. Learning how to say, "No," would be a good place to start.

A word of warning, not all medications are for all people. Some anti-depressants can have very adverse effects: some are addictive, and a lot just mask what the real problem is. Don't hesitate to speak up if you think your loved one is being over-medicated or is not doing well on a drug. In some cases, a drug that has helped the patient for two years can become ineffective and even start causing bad side effects.

Some of the patients from nursing homes that come in for eye examinations are over-medicated. They are just like zombies, with slurred speech. They are barely able to hold their heads up, much less read the chart. It is a pathetic, heart-rending sight. This may be necessary in certain cases where the patient is constantly very agitated or aggressive, however, when over-medication is done for the convenience of the caregivers in the facility, I get very angry and upset.

PSYCHOLOGISTS . . . there are psychologists, and then there are psychologists. According to Webster's, a psychologist is a specialist in the scientific study of the mental and behavioral characteristics of a person or group. As with finding the right psychiatrist, it is important to find the right psychologist to help in dealing with someone's personal insecurities, negative thinking and/or depression.

Hindsight is always better than foresight, but looking back, I wish now that my husband had seen a psychologist. He masked his feelings and problems with heavy-duty drugs given by a psychiatrist. What he needed was to work through his grief for his brother, who died tragically in a plane crash. He needed to learn how to face the problems that life had dealt him. If he had, he might not have needed me as his caregiver for the rest of his life.

Mental health is a critical part of caring for a disabled person. If you think taking your loved one to a psychiatrist or a psychologist could possibly improve your dependent's quality of life, do so now. It could make looking back a lot less painful.

Q

QUALITY OF LIFE for the dependent is always a concern. The caring caregiver is always looking for ways to improve the dependent's comfort and participation in daily events. The problem with this scenario is that, in the process, you tend to overlook the need for quality in your own life. It is just as important for you to be actively enjoying life and growing. You need your own personal diversions. See Hobbies under "H."

When the quality of life has deteriorated to the point that the physical body of the dependent is barely functioning and in great pain, it's time to let go. The ill person often controls the decision as to when.

The "will to live" is very powerful in the human spirit. Our brother-in-law, Dave, was dying of cancer. I think he would have died a few months before he actually did, but he had promised his daughter he would walk her down the aisle when she got married. The wedding was several months away. Dave was determined to make it because he knew how much it meant to her. The bride was radiant, but I'll never forget seeing the presence of death in that brave father's face as he walked his daughter down the aisle.

Janice Hucknall Snyder

He supported himself on the side panel of each pew. He had kept his promise. He even danced one dance with his daughter at the reception before he went home and back to bed. But, that isn't the end of the story of Dave's strong will. A few days later, Dave's robust brother, who had sadly watched Dave in his walk down the aisle, dropped dead. He had a massive heart attack. Dave arose from his bed one more time. He insisted on being driven two-and-a-half hours to attend his brother's funeral. Then he went home and passed away quietly a week later. His love of family and his courage will live in my memory the rest of my days.

Someone else I will never forget is a patient we had who was ninety-four. She was almost bent in half with Osteoporosis. She looked up at me with a pained expression and said, "I think God has forgotten about me." Thankfully, He remembered a few months later.

QUANTITY BUYING is the smart way to go. It saves money, time and gasoline. Check prices and shop at the large wholesale marts. There are drawbacks, though. Quantity buying requires larger money output all at one time and more storage space. Plus, the packaging will be bulkier and heavier. I solved the weight problem with my dishwasher soap and some food products, such as coffee and jam, by transferring part of the contents to smaller, lightweight plastic containers. It saves in the lifting department. Every bit helps.

QUARRELLING is unpleasant, at best. Some ill people can be downright quarrelsome. No matter what you do or say, they want to complain and fuss. It is unpleasant to listen to, day in and day out. Quarreling is a negative, and it is hard on one's patience.

One poor soul was in our office just today. She complained that the bathroom for the patients was too small for her with her walker. "Don't you have another bathroom that is bigger?" she whined. I told her there was a larger bathroom for the employees that she was welcome to use. Showing her the way, I listened to her quarrelsome voice complaining that it was an awfully long way to go. When she finally got there, she looked and said, "Well, this is small too."

By then, my patience was waning, so I said, "This bathroom is three times the size of the other one. Do you want to use it or not?" She used it. I could tell by the look on the caregiver's face that she was having a miserable time trying to manage this unpleasant person.

I am fortunate that this kind of problem for the caregiver is not mine. But if it were, I would be very firm with this type of person. I would not reply to a whining, complaining, quarrelsome individual. I would ask him/her to repeat what was being said in a nice, mannerly way if an answer was expected from me. Firmness and consistency are important in handling this kind of problem if the caregiver wants to keep from going bonkers. The need to discipline an adult person seems unnatural, but as with small children, if the caregiver doesn't keep control, they lose it. That's not a good situation in any case. It's hard on survival.

Quarreling, between the caregiver and the patient, is always very upsetting to both. It's best to resolve disagreements as quickly as possible because of the emotional upheaval they can cause between two people who are so connected by their circumstances. The caregiver should keep in control of the situation, compromising with the patient in order to ease the dilemma when appropriate.

QUESTIONS produce answers and answers broaden your learning, no matter what the subject. I always had trouble asking questions. I was afraid the person I was asking would think I was dumb because my question was. I'm sure this fear was the result of asking a "stupid" question in class when I was young and having the whole class, including the teacher, laugh and make fun of me. After that, it was a long time before I risked asking another question, which was my loss. I finally reached the age where what other people thought of silly questions, or anything else, didn't bother me. Hurrah for me. I hope you learned this lesson quicker than I did.

There are all kinds of people in this world; some like to intimidate others. Brilliant doctors don't always have a good "bedside manner." There are doctors who talk over your head or talk very rapidly because they have had to say the same things over and over again, daily. Most people are just naturally nervous when visiting the doctor. That is why it helps to have your questions ready and written down. If you don't understand the doctor's answer, tell him so. If he acts annoyed and hurries you, find another doctor if your insurance allows it. There are many doctors out there who are just as good, or even better. Find a doctor with patience and understanding; someone willing to take the time to explain the best way to deal with the problems you are facing. You should be able to ask all the questions you want, even the dumb ones. Anything you can learn to help you care for your patient also helps you to survive the caring.

QUIET TIME, my kingdom for some quiet time! Ah, the blessed relief of having time to yourself. Take advantage of every chance you get to have this kind of time. It is a time for meditation and renewal of inner strength, both so important in keeping the caregiver going. Set aside a certain time each day just for you. Make the time, even if it means setting the alarm clock fifteen minutes earlier in the morning or staying up fifteen minutes later at night. Recharge so you won't discharge the wrong words on others.

QUITTING, you might think, should not be a word in the caregiver's vocabulary for survival. This book is all about how to manage, not quit. Wrong! If you get to the point where your own survival is in jeopardy, it is time to quit. Some of the things that could make you reach this point are personal medical problems, your own symptoms of a nervous breakdown, exhaustion, danger from uncontrollable, violent outbursts from your patient, etc. If any of these are the case, then quit you must, to survive. This may be accomplished by turning your duties as caregiver over to another relative (or relatives), or it may be time to make the difficult judgment to transfer your loved one to a nursing home. Don't wait until it is too late. Where your wellbeing is concerned, don't allow your heart to overrule your good judgment in making a timely decision.

Janice Hucknall Snyder

R

READING is a wonderful pastime and escape for the caregiver. It transports you to anywhere else for a brief respite from the worries and responsibilities of the day. An accessible library makes it a zero expense, unless you're one of those people who are always late returning books. Some people only read one or two types of books. I don't see how they can limit themselves like that when there is such a wonderful variety in reading to be experienced. Oh well, to each his own. The important thing is for you to enjoy this diversion, since you are tied down with caregiver duties.

Does your loved one stay in a day-care center while you hold down a full-time job? Then you may be too busy and tired at night to do much reading. CD tapes are the answer. They are wonderful. You can listen to audiobooks while driving back and forth to work each day. My round trip driving time is one hour. About once a week I go to the library and check out three audio books. I'm so busy enjoying the stories, I don't get impatient with bad drivers and traffic problems. If you are lucky enough to be just a few minutes from your office, you could still enjoy this form of entertainment in your home. Give your eyes a rest. The person you are caring for might enjoy listening too.

REALITY is what the caregiver and the ill person have to face as the stages of the disease advance, affecting the quality of life of the loved one. Hospice is a wonderful group of caring people who help those who are facing the reality of dying. They assist the caregiver in giving medications for the relief of suffering. The many people I know who have received help from Hospice have had only praise for the benefits and support the Hospice program provided them. Your doctor is the best person to determine when it is time to request Hospice.

RECEPTIVENESS to the mental and physical needs of the dependent is vital for their wellbeing. Sometimes patients mask their true feelings when contemplating suicide. Sometimes they are unable to communicate a physical problem to you. Keep the lines of communication open. Discuss everything under the sun on a regular basis. That way you are better able to stay acutely aware of and receptive to changes in mood.

When you are dedicated to the needs of your loved one, you may find little time to be receptive to your own feelings and physical needs. Don't let this happen to you. Take time to ask yourself how you are doing and give honest answers (yes, it's okay to talk to yourself). Remember, just as you have to love yourself before you are able to love others, so too, you have to feel whole to have the strength to care well for another. It is a vital part of your survival.

RECONCILING rifts in relationships requires restraint and reason. When you keep your self-control and communicate fairness in understanding the other person's viewpoint, the door is left open for reconciliation.

Disagreements, whether with your dependent or another family member, put a terrible burden on your emotions. The distress a break in a relationship can cause can actually lower your resistance to physical ailments. Don't let a day go by wherein you have not dealt in a positive way with any conflict of personalities.

RECORDS are a necessary pain in the neck. Keeping track of such things as medical expenses, drugs, dates of physical exams, physical changes, I.R.S. data, household expenses, etc., is another one of those duties that has to be handled with some sort of regularity and order.

I have a file cabinet filled with alphabetical folders covering every expense. This works well for me and eases the burden of this time consuming task. The more details put into my record keeping, the better able I am to figure out what I need to later on. This is especially important with anything relating to medical expenses for my husband. Find a filing system that works for you and keep up with it. When records pile up, they tend to get mislaid and are much harder to put in proper order. If you have a computer, you can put the important facts there, but be certain to back it up. It is a time-consuming task, regardless. The better organized you are, the less time this task will take and the less hair you'll pull out.

Keep a record of changes in your patient's condition. It's easy to forget. Such things as fluctuations in mood and when the effectiveness of medications wears off are of vital interest to the doctor. These statistics help him to determine the dosage and strength of medications and whether or not changes in medication are needed. Your job is easier when your loved one is kept at comfortable levels.

REGRETS are something all of us have from time to time. We regret opportunities not acted on, wrong decisions made, unkind words spoken, mistaken judgments, etc. As a caregiver, you are bound to have regrets in the handling of your loved one. The stress and emotional involvement make you very vulnerable. When you are tired and feeling bad, your level of patience will be at a low point. Don't be too hard on yourself. Remember you have feelings and failings, just like everyone else. Dwelling on regrets can be devastating to your morale. Blaming yourself excessively can lead to depression and feelings of failure. Stop those kinds of thoughts before they take hold of you. Draw from happy experiences, not regrets.

Some people use their regrets as a crutch their whole lives through. Have you ever known someone who was always saying, "If only this or that hadn't happened," or "If only I had done so and so?" Expressing regrets about your current situation or looking for sympathy all the time doesn't make for good company, and caregivers need good company to help them survive.

RELATIONSHIPS can only develop and last if the two people involved share the four Ls: love, loyalty, laughter and listening. These four Ls are important in a marriage. These same four Ls are important in the relationship between you, the caregiver, and the person you are caring for. Without any one of them, your relationship can become crippled; then caring becomes a burden. Actively work at keeping the four Ls alive and well with your dependent. You will be glad you did.

RELATIVES, if you've treated them right, are a wonderful asset. If you haven't, quick, read what I wrote about in "FORGIVENESS" and start getting back in their good graces.

My husband and I have been blessed with a very loving, caring family. All four of our children live within fifteen miles of our home, which is great. We have the added good fortune of having three super sons-in-law and one lovely daughter-in-law. All in all, they have been very supportive and helpful in keeping us going. Even our three teenage grandsons have looked after their "Pop Pop" while I made a dash to the store.

I hope you have lots of family members you can call on to help at times. Do it on a regular basis to give yourself needed breaks. For instance, if you have four capable relatives living nearby, delegate each of them one week of the month. Then have them pick one day in that week that they will be available for you for three hours. If the person works, then an evening or Saturday or Sunday will do. I don't think you will have any trouble finding people who would gladly give three hours a month to help out. You can do a variety of things in three hours: see a movie, eat dinner out, go for a swim, visit friends, or even go to bed and catch up on your sleep. These special hours would be something for you to look forward to every week. You know who else would feel good about this? Your "good-deeders," that's who.

RELAXING is what the caregiver could always do more of. It seems like the minute I sit down to rest and unwind, I suddenly remember it's time to give my husband his medication, or the phone rings, or someone stops by, or it's time to start dinner, or-or-or.

So I catch what moments I can, and when I'm smart, I don't answer the phone at all. I do listen to the recording on the answering machine, though, in case it's terribly important. Nothing is more irritating than having the phone ring while you're trying to relax or eat dinner, unless it's finding a solicitor on the other end of the phone line requesting money. Do whatever it takes to keep from being interrupted while having a few precious moments of repose. Don't hesitate to let others know it's time for them to do a disappearing act.

REMINISCING about past happy events with someone who has memory loss can be a stimulating experience for the both of you. I have discovered that even when my husband can't tell me my name or who I am, if I start telling him about something special or funny that happened to us years ago, he smiles and even comments on the event. In keeping with this, I have started getting out the old photo albums to show him again (both of us being photography nuts, there are over sixty albums). These are enjoyable ways of connecting that you and your loved one can share. Memories stay special for a lifetime.

REPRESSING emotions all the time is not good for survival. Just as a teakettle has to let off steam with a whistle, so too, the caregiver has to release built up pressure. There are many different ways you can do this. Find what way works best for you. Talking to a sympathetic listener, crying, screaming, taking hot showers, writing, dancing, exercising and masturbating have all been discussed in this book as ways to relieve stress. The main thing is to recognize the need before you blow your top, or someone else's.

RESPONSIBILITIES can be overwhelming for the caregiver. Caring for the ill person is responsibility enough, but every phase of existence is laid on your shoulders. It is a long list: handling financial matters, supplying staples, repairing the home, cleaning the house and clothes, recycling garbage, yard work, preparing meals and even holding down a full-time job to meet expenses. How do you do all of these things? Sometimes you just don't. You do the best that you can. You don't fret if it doesn't all get done.

Accept outside help whenever it's offered. Don't be a martyr. Don't be shy. You are trying to survive awesome responsibilities.

REWARDS are something the caregiver deserves. And how! You should give yourself rewards on a regular basis. Whether it's big or small, having something kind of special to look forward to is what's important. It's even fun to try to think of things that are different, like an outing to a museum, a bike ride on the beach, a banana split, buying a favorite movie, getting a pedicure, etc. This concept works well for the dependent too. Everyone needs fun things to look forward to.

RUSHING is unavoidable at times, especially for the caregiver who is holding down a full-time job. Rushing all the time, however, is a no-no. Something has to give before you give out. Analyze everything being done. Cut down on non-essentials. Check the efficiency of routine procedures. Combine tasks that can be done simultaneously. For instance, while keeping an eye on the cake that is baking, clean out the refrigerator and make the grocery list. Time saved is time earned. Time earned gives you more time to do other chores at an unhurried pace, or better still, gives you more time to relax. Make yourself slow down. Sometimes, we hurry, hurry, hurry out of habit. Then, we're frazzled, frazzled, frazzled all the time. This could lead to shingles, high blood pressure, migraine, heart attack, or stroke and, of course, mental and physical exhaustion. Are those enough side effects to scare you? They should be. They don't do much for survival either.

Janice Hucknall Snyder

SACRIFICING is certainly a part of what the caregiver's life is all about. A lot is given up for the sake of another.

A young black man came into our office recently, sent by MEPS (Military Entrance Processing Station). The military wanted his eye problem evaluated before accepting him into the service. He was very worried that he wouldn't be accepted. In talking to him, I found out he had been a caregiver to his diabetic mother for the past nine years, since he was fourteen years old. All of his brothers and sisters had deserted him. He had just now put his mother in a nursing home. He said, "I can't take care of her any longer. I feel guilty, but I just have to start living my own life." I told him that after giving nine years of his youth caring for his mother, he had no reason to feel guilty. She should want him to have a life of his own after the sacrifices he had made. We hear so many negative "newsworthy" stories about teenagers. I was deeply touched and impressed with the courage of this fine young man. He made my day.

All caregivers need to know there are limits to how much of themselves they can sacrifice for another. When the caring stops being given lovingly and starts being given grudgingly, it's time to pull back. Make some schedule changes that allow more time for you. Even if it is only a few extra hours a week, it will be significant to you. The loss of the freedom to come and go whenever, wherever and for however long one wants is the biggest sacrifice of all.

SCHEDULES are a necessary pain in the neck. Nevertheless, they are important from the standpoint that, without a schedule, everything is utter chaos. Nothing gets completed when it should, which adds to the pressure. But schedules shouldn't be so important that one runs over ten people trying to keep them. Scheduling, done in moderation (as so many things should be), is bound to make your day go more smoothly.

SECLUSION is hard to come by when one is a caregiver. You need a place of seclusion where you can meditate. Spending a quiet hour alone is a wonderful way to renew the spirit, which is your source of energy.

SELF-CONTROL when lost, doesn't usually return before causing regrets. People who lose their self-control quickly when angry are said to have a "short fuse." One does not want to be anywhere near "short fuses" when they explode.

Caregivers need a lot of self-control in dealing with a dependent who is being unpleasant. But don't let the patient get away with being rude without responding to the issue. Let the patient know that unkind remarks make you feel bad. If you say unkind, hurtful things yourself, it usually makes things worse; there are regrets later. Remember to be thankful you are not the patient.

Survival of the Caregiver

SELF-ESTEEM is one of the most important words in this book. Individuals usually don't talk about their self-esteem. Most people's self-esteem is so low they wouldn't care to discuss it anyway. Webster's says self-esteem means "one's good opinion of one's dignity or worth." In order to be perfectly clear, I also looked up the word dignity. The dictionary explains dignity as "insisting on being treated with respect." Now that gets to the crux of the matter. Anyone wanting to be treated with respect (and most of us really would like to be) must value his/her own self-worth in order to feel deserving of that consideration. People who let others "walk all over them," even beat them up, "don't get any respect."

I know of a lady who is a Beauty Consultant. Her expertise is in "making over" women. They seek her services because they want to improve their appearance. They want to make a better impression in the business world and in their personal contacts. This consultant teaches them the correct colors to use, how to coordinate their clothing, hair styling, and the right shades of makeup and how to apply them, etc. When she is finished, they look like a million dollars and are thrilled with their new image. The sad thing about this scenario is that, six months later, the makeover artist will see many of these same customers again. They will be back to the way they looked when they first came in. This is because no matter how you fancy up the outside, if there is no self-esteem inside, the characteristics of low self-esteem re-surface. They arrive in the form of apathy and a lack of incentive to keep up a good appearance. Plastic surgeons recognize this. In order for their patients to be happy with the results of surgery, the patients must already feel good and secure about themselves.

So what has this got to do with being a caregiver? Plenty! When you have self-esteem, you value your life. You feel deserving of any enjoyment that can be had, even while caring for another. This gives balance to your life and goes a long way in helping you to survive. Without self-esteem, the caregiver doesn't feel worthy of pleasure. Should something fun happen to cross his/her path, no doubt, feelings of guilt will follow.

SELFISHNESS is often a trait in young children. Too bad many never outgrow it. Is it selfish for the caregiver to enjoy activities that the totally confined dependent cannot? Of course not! You need stimulations that will keep you in a good frame of mind and keep you physically healthy. This is an advantage to the confined person as well. When you feel good, quite naturally, you will do a better job of caring for the dependent. Selfishness should not be a word in the caregiver's vocabulary. It can seep into your thinking, closely followed by the word guilt. Both words are destructive to your wellbeing.

SHARING feelings with others who are dealing with similar problems is helpful. This type of interaction is very supportive and a lot cheaper than a psychiatrist. There are support group meetings for alcoholics, widows, single parents, dieters, compulsive gamblers, and drug addicts, and of course, for all the major illnesses, such as cancer, Parkinson's, depression, muscular dystrophy, diabetes and multiple sclerosis, to name a few.

If you are not "group" oriented, that's okay. But everyone needs at least one other person they can unload on, or they will burst and come apart at the seams. Negative thoughts and feelings that keep building up inside have to get out or they will eat away at your very being. They erode your thinking, causing mental and physical problems. So share your feelings. It's good for healing.

Survival of the Caregiver

When your mate is ill with Alzheimer's disease, or another form of dementia, sharing is one of the things you miss the most. My husband and I shared thoughts about our children and what we believed in. We shared feelings and supported one another. We shared compliments and jokes, happiness and sorrow, aches and pains, dreams and goals, and love, hugs and kisses. That sharing is deeply missed. No wonder there is a sense of great loss long before death occurs.

SHATTERED is the name of a poignant song Linda Ronstadt sings. Something that is shattered is broken into pieces. The caregiver's life is shattered, altered forever, by the catastrophic illness of a loved one. The enormity of the change can be overwhelming at times. Our hearts feel shattered and broken as well. We cannot put the pieces back together again like a jigsaw puzzle. We cannot make the picture of our lives look like it did before ever again.

We can grow closer in our relationships with the other people we love, though. We can also develop a new awareness of the true value and meaning of life. This is a different kind of picture, but it has value too.

SHOES are for walking. If you couldn't complain until after you had walked a mile in another man's shoes, you probably wouldn't complain at all. The point is, when you get to feeling sorry for yourself, you should think about how much worse the ill person's life must be. The real horror is being helpless and having to rely on another human being, all the time, for every need. Those are shoes no one wants to wear; be thankful they are not on your feet.

SHOPPING is a dreaded drudgery or a fun-filled spree. It all depends on how much money is in the wallet and what's on the shopping list. I stay away from department stores as much as possible. When I walk through those swinging doors, I leave all my willpower behind in the parking lot. I rationalize about all kinds of things I didn't know I needed until now. Of course, each item is a bargain, marked down at least three times. This is a costly weakness, so I mostly stick to the drudgery of buying essentials like food, depends, toothpaste, depends, plastic items, depends, cleaning products and more depends. Again, as mentioned elsewhere, always buy items in large quantities. It cuts down on the time and energy expended, as well as cost and temptation.

SHOWERS are a daily respite mentioned in other areas of this book as a means of relieving tension, relaxing aching muscles, etc. It's a place to not only cleanse the body, but also to cleanse the cluttered mind of unwanted feelings of anger and despair. A long soak in a hot tub is mighty fine for this purpose too. Cold showers should not be over-looked though. In hot weather, cold showers are invigorating and get the tired blood circulating. They revive and refresh, aiding you in surviving and facing the rigors of yet another day.

SING in the rain, snow or sunshine. Sing when you're sad or mad, sing in the shower or the car, but sing. It's great for lifting your spirits and exercising your lungs. It's just a fun thing to do. I sing while driving to and from work, especially the latter. I used to get strange looks from other drivers who thought I was talking to myself. Now, with so many people using car phones, I "appear" normal. It doesn't matter that you can't carry a tune, if you're alone that is (a listening friend with perfect pitch could be lost forever). Don't worry. If you don't remember all the words, fake it or hum, but use those vocal cords.

Survival of the Caregiver

SLEEPING is easier said than done at times. A caregiver has to deal with a lot of stress and worry, two factors that are no help at all in sleeping. Some nights you just can't get to sleep. Other times you wake up in the middle of the night. I keep a boring book handy that usually does the trick. Sleeping pills are a no, no, and should be used only as a last resort, and maybe not even then. They can be habit-forming, and people often end up needing to increase the dosage for effectiveness. Eventually, pills decrease your effectiveness, so find other ways to get those "ZZZs," such as: drinking warm milk, listening to soft music or subliminal tapes, reading, watching TV, praying; whatever turns you off. The main thing is to relax your body and empty your mind of worrisome thoughts. Use whatever method works best and fastest for you. A good eight or nine hours of sleep is essential for you to stay healthy and alert.

SMILE and the whole world smiles with you, frown and you frown alone. There is a lot of truth in that old saying, which I've butchered a bit to fit this subject. Caregivers take note: people who always look like they have a chip on their shoulder and never smile (even though they may have good reason not to), are not fun to be with or live with.

I smile a lot, mostly because my face looks so awful when I'm not smiling. Without a smile, my eyes and mouth sag and I look ten years older. That's the truth. There is a more important reason why I smile though. It makes me feel better and lifts my spirits. I look for the humor in daily happenings to smile and laugh about. It keeps me going.

The comics in the newspaper are always good for a smile. I remember asking my tennis partner if she had read a particularly funny strip I'd seen in the paper that morning. She looked at me like I was crazy and said, "I never read the funnies." I was aghast. (That's a little dramatic, but I was.)

I replied, "Really? I thought everyone read the comics."

Her next remark was even more startling. She said, "I've never found the funnies very funny." The following month, I cut out and saved all the "extra funny" strips. I mailed a fat envelope of them to her. I was rewarded with a phone call. "Yes, they really were funny," she admitted. I smiled.

Sometimes it is hard to smile when things aren't going well. Try faking a big smile for a while, it could trick your brain into thinking you feel happy. Then you'll start feeling better, and the smile will be for real.

SMOKE ALARMS are inexpensive, easy to install and can give you the time you need to escape a burning house. If your loved one is disabled, you need all the time you can get. Install alarms on each floor level of your home and in every bedroom, storage space and hallway. Directions come with them to tell you where the placement should be. Be sure to check them on a regular basis. Make sure the battery is alive and well so you will be too. Keep a supply of the type battery required on hand. When the battery gets low in some smoke alarms, they start beeping to let you know. One late night, four different alarms started beeping at about the same time. I didn't have any replacements on hand. I had to remove the weak batteries so I could get my ZZZs.

Have a plan for different escape routes, depending on the placement of smoke and flames. Call 911 first, if you can reach a phone. Don't open a hot door; do stay close to the floor. Keep a fire extinguisher on each floor and know how to use it.

SOLUTIONS to problems can be as close as the nose on your face. So often I've taken the long way around to find the right answer. Some of the biggest problems have the simplest solutions. I'll fret and worry over something for a long time. Finally, I'll give up and put it out of my mind. Then the answer will come to me suddenly, out of the blue. It still amazes me when that happens. Any method that cuts down on worrying is worth trying.

I was in the habit of fixing my husband and I breakfast first thing in the morning after we were dressed. Then I'd curl my hair, put on cosmetics and do other chores before leaving for work. This was difficult because of the need to keep checking on my husband. One morning, I broke the habit. I changed the routine. It finally occurred to me to shower my husband and put him back to bed until everything I had to do was done. It was a breeze. I finished in half the time. Then I got Richard up and dressed, and we had a much more leisurely breakfast. The solution was simple, worked well and was a lot easier on both of us.

I just recently discovered a great solution to the problem of having wet sheets in the morning, but it wasn't my solution. The nursing director at the facility where Dick stays during the day gave it to me. She said to put two diapers on the patient at bedtime, cutting a slit in the bottom area of the first diaper so that the excess can go through and be absorbed in the second diaper. Wish I'd thought of that two years ago. It sure would have saved a lot of washing and extra work.

If you don't let yourself get too set in your way of doing things, you are more apt to come up with solutions for doing them better.

SPIRIT is at the center of our very being. It is a holy power that gives us the strength and will to do all the good that we do. Without it, I am nothing. Without spirit, there is no way I could fulfill my part as a caregiver. There is no way I could face problems and find energy, day in and day out. Without my inner spirit, there is no way I could survive.

Tap into your spirit; be aware that it is there for you. Draw power from your spirit through prayer and meditation. It will sustain you when there is a need.

STRESS, who needs it? No one. Who gets it? Everyone. Life is full of situations that create stress. Family conflicts, pressures on the job, health problems, car breakdowns and heavy debts all take a toll. To top it off, it isn't unusual to have several sources of stress going on simultaneously. That's when we have to look out, because our stress factor is on "overload." Caregivers are very vulnerable to this kind of overload. Unless the stress is defused, health problems can develop.

I have discussed several ways to relieve stress in other parts of this book, under "EXERCISE," "VACATIONS," "HOBBIES," and "INTERCOURSE." So in this segment, I'm listing some very easy, basic exercises for stress. They can be done just about anywhere, some even in the car while waiting at a red light. Don't grit your teeth while doing these. Relax. Say to yourself, "I'm in control" (even if you don't think you are).

- Do each movement 10 times.
- Rotate eyes slowly, clockwise then counter clockwise.
- Rotate the neck slowly, clockwise then counter clockwise.
- Rotate shoulders forward slowly, then backwards, then up and down.

- Hug yourself, stretch your arms up, hug again, stretch arms forward, hug once more, and stretch arms sideways.
- Open and close fists, stroke each finger, touch thumbs to each finger.
- Rotate feet clockwise, then counter clockwise, then move them up and down.
- Pull knees up to chest with your arms around them. Hold to the count of ten. (This one is not too easy in the car, especially if you are driving.)

Other ways of relieving stress are Biofeedback, Yoga and Transcendental Meditation, all of which require instruction and serious study. On a smaller scale, try talking to yourself, saying things like, "My hands are warm," "The air is cool," or, "My body is relaxed." (I wouldn't recommend doing this where anyone could notice; they might not understand.)

SUCCESS is how one perceives it. Is success the most important thing in your life? A lot of people think so and work eighteen-hour days to achieve it. Some make it and some don't. Some destroy their health or die trying. If success is the most important thing in a person's life, failure can be devastating and followed by a heart attack, stroke, breakdown or suicide. Perhaps too much importance is placed on the need to succeed.

Recently, a patient came in for his eye examination and announced, "I'm going to be 94 tomorrow," adding, "Look how great I look!" I had to agree, and his mental capacity was sharp as a tack. I asked him what he owed his longevity to. He replied, "I have always been concerned about being happy, rather than successful. If you do things in your life that make you a happy person, you will usually be a successful person too. People that think success is making a million dollars may or may not succeed in reaching that goal. But if they do reach it, do you know what they want then? They want another million. They want power. They are never satisfied." The patient who made this astute observation is a retired doctor, a wise old one.

As a caregiver, it is equally important to strive to be happy in your daily life and keep a good attitude. I hope you are successful at doing that. Life is precious, to be savored, no matter what the circumstances.

SUICIDE is a scary word and terribly hard to deal with. In every life it touches, it leaves deep, painful scars. Suicide affects every family member, relative and friend that the individual knew. I mentioned suicide briefly under "DEPRESSION" because that condition is where the seeds for suicide begin. The pain of depression is more severe than a lot of physical illnesses. It can be caused by the loss of a loved one, loss of a job, financial ruin, retirement, inherited genetics and even certain medications. It also causes other serious physical illnesses such as cancer, arthritis and heart disease. It breaks down the immune system, which is so vital to good health. Depression causes suicide, so don't waste any time in getting help against this silent killer. If your loved one (or you yourself) is experiencing symptoms of depression, seek help immediately. Find a competent doctor. Keeping a distressed person alive until the crisis has passed is what survival is all about.

SUPPORTIVE is what we should all be more of with each other. It is one of the most important attributes parents can have when raising their children. In our desire to have "good kids" we tend to give our children "constructive" criticism about everything, with a few supportive pats on the back thrown in along the way. It should be the other way around. I was guilty of this; just ask my first-born.

A lot of children put other kids down every chance they get; making fun of others is a big game. I often ask patients when they got their first pair of glasses. Many say that they were between the ages of six to sixteen, and then they add, "But I only wore them two or three months; I couldn't take the teasing." They preferred to see the world as a blur, rather than be heckled by their insensitive peers.

When I was twelve, my brother, Jack, was sixteen. He was always trying to compose songs and would sing them to me, wanting my approval. Naturally, I always said they were no good, just to tease. Supportive, I was not. Sibling rivalry, you know. One day, Jack cornered me and said he had new lyrics and music for a song he just knew could be a smash hit. With that, he burst into song. When finished, he said, "Well, what do you think, Janice? Isn't it great?"

I gave a shrug and said, "Well, Jack, it could be worse, but no way would it ever be a hit." He burst out laughing and told me it wasn't really his song. Jack smugly informed me that it was already a big hit. The song was Blowin in the Wind by Bob Dylan. I guess he showed me. I've learned to be a much more supportive person since then.

Caregivers need others to be supportive of them while they are being supportive of the dependent. A lot of people are so busy "supporting" themselves, achieving their own goals and dealing with the problems of their own lives (we all have them), that they don't have time to be concerned for others. It's called selfishness. Mature people outgrow this condition and have much happier lives once "I" isn't the most used letter in their vocabulary. My husband and I have been blessed with very supportive people in our lives. No wonder I'm surviving.

Janice Hucknall Snyder

T

TACT is something I probably shouldn't be writing about, because I'm not qualified. I tend to be outspoken. Thinking before I speak is not one of my attributes; how I wish it were. I am trying to improve in this department, but I still say things that would be a lot better left unsaid.

Although tact isn't anything that really affects your survival, there was a day and age when saying something out of line could mean a challenge to a duel which only one would survive. It's a good thing I didn't live back then. Sometimes people will ask tactless questions about your ill person. If it is something you would rather not discuss, just say so in a "tactful" way.

TEETH can become a problem in a patient who has any form of dementia. Sometimes they regurgitate, and this can increase the chances of decay. The caregiver has to take over the responsibility of making sure teeth are cleaned properly. Our dentist advised using an electric brush to facilitate the job. It does make it easier for you to clean teeth well. Check with your dentist to see which type of toothpaste he thinks is most suitable for your loved one.

Janice Hucknall Snyder

It is difficult to clean someone else's teeth, but it needs to be done after breakfast and dinner. Use a gum stimulator or a proxabrush to get in between the teeth where food gets caught and decays. Be careful to stay clear of the teeth if you don't want to lose a finger.

TELEPHONES should be in key places to save you extra steps. Portable phones and cell phones are great. If I'm on the phone and my husband gets up and wanders out of the room, I can keep right on talking while following after him. An answering machine, either in the home or with a service on line, is also a great asset. You won't miss important messages if tied up with caring for your loved one. Better still, when a salesperson is on the line, you can avoid the call completely. This is especially satisfying at dinnertime because that is when they always call no matter what time you eat.

TELEVISION is a great pastime for the disabled. My husband always loved to play golf, so he thoroughly enjoys watching all of the tournaments. TV is a wonderful diversion for you, too. Besides regular programming, the educational channel on Cable has a variety of continuing education programs to stimulate your interest. If you don't use your brain, you lose it. More important, when you are listening and learning, you have less time to dwell on how restricted your life has become, which is a real downer if you do dwell on it.

TEMPERS need tempering. Everyone knows what it is like to be around someone with a bad temper, someone who flies off the handle easily. Stay clear of that type of person as much as possible. Who needs that kind of unpleasantness? It is especially unhealthy to be around someone who is inclined to throw things. If your patient has a temper that puts you under added stress, just what you don't need, it is important to handle this type of situation calmly, but firmly. Do not hesitate to seek help from a psychiatrist or your family doctor if the problem becomes uncontrollable.

If you, yourself, have a temper, try to avoid situations that you know will make you angry. For example, you know you lose your temper when someone makes you late for an appointment. You also know your dependent does things that cause delays. By adding fifteen minutes to the time allowed for getting ready, you maintain control of the situation and are able to keep your cool.

Tempers usually flare when people are over-tired, tense or worried about something. Of course, these are all familiar conditions you deal with as a caregiver.

TIME is the most precious gift you are given in life, and no one knows just what his/her allotment will be. You should use your share fully and wisely.

When I was twenty-two, a very important and good thing happened to me. I almost died in childbirth. The doctors couldn't get my pulse for two hours; it was so weak. That experience changed my attitude about life completely, and for the better. I had always worried about every little thing. Not anymore. Of course, I worry if someone I love is critically ill, but the greatest gift I got from my close call with death was an appreciation for life. I have wasted very little of it ever since. I fill each day to the fullest with diverse activities. No matter how much has to be done at work and at home for my dependent, I always make sure I do something that is just for me. When the sand in the hourglass runs out, I will have no regrets. I made sure I did all the important things I wanted to do in my life as I went along. Have you? I am very thankful that I got that second chance forty-three years ago. Appreciate the fragility of life, and make the most of each day that is given to you.

TIREDNESS goes hand in hand with being a caregiver. It is very tedious, mentally and physically, to care for a disabled person. Need I tell you? But, if you feel tired out all the time, even when getting proper rest, which is a warning sign that should be taken seriously. It could be caused by a number of things: anemia, depression, stress, high blood pressure, or other medical problems. Check with your doctor, before it becomes a fight for your own survival.

TOUCHING is a contact that has more meaning then any words can convey. In certain situations, when it is difficult to find words, touching is a way of expressing yourself. It is a tender way to communicate. Touching, between the caregiver and the ill person, is an important means of expressing feeling. It keeps the bond of caring warm and alive. It gives a good feeling; something both of you can always use more of.

TRAVELING, at best, is a tedious ordeal. When the dependent is mobile and there is a need to travel by plane, you have your hands full. Recently, my husband's mom turned ninety-years-old. The immediate family decided to celebrate by giving her a big birthday party. Fifty-six relatives, including great-grandchildren, descended on Summit, New Jersey. It was a very special reunion that none of us will ever forget. I worried a lot about how the traveling would go. I was pleasantly surprised with the accommodations available. I didn't know you could call ahead and have a wheelchair waiting for you at your destination, so we had to wait a few minutes for one. When the chair arrived, the person bringing it took charge of wheeling my husband down to baggage claim. That was very helpful. The only problem I had was fitting the two of us into the tiny bathroom on the plane. Since I'm 5' 9", and my husband is 6', that was a real challenge. The expressions on the passengers' faces when we came out together were well worth the effort, though. I could hardly keep a straight face.

If at all possible, don't limit yourselves to just car travel. Travel and change are good, so be brave and plan well ahead.

TRUST is earned through actions taken that prove a person's reliability and sincerity. A true, trusted friend is to be cherished during one's lifetime. When you are a caregiver, a trusted friend is indeed a blessing. It is someone you can count on to support you when you are down. It is someone you can share your feelings with. I pray you have someone like that to hold hands with.

It is also important for you to be worthy of trust from the ill person you are caring for. Your dependent relies on you for his/her every need. Trust brings a feeling of security to a helpless person. When the ill person feels secure, he/she is less anxious and, therefore, easier to handle. Completing the circle, when things are easier to handle for you, it improves your chances for survival. Trust me.

TRY. Just try. That's the least anyone can do. The word "can't" should be deleted from the dictionary. Again, it's the difference between thinking positively and negatively. Now that my husband is unable to do any repairs around the house, I've had to learn to "fix" things. We bought a house built in 1917. Over the years, we have both done a lot of painting, wallpapering, repairing, etc., so I'm no stranger to a hammer, screwdriver or saw. This made the transition easier for me. When our son and sons-in-law come to visit, they are always great about fixing what I've tried and been unable to handle. Husbands with disabled wives have to learn to cook, do laundry, shop, etc. A lot of men are already experts at barbecuing, so that's a good start, although I've never tried a barbecued egg. There will be failures, of course, but at least there are many pre-prepared dinners you can buy to keep from starving. "Do It Yourself" books help in areas where you are a novice. I've found that employees in hardware stores are very helpful and nice about showing me how the thing-a-ma-jig fits into the what-cha-ma-call-it on my dishwasher. Keep trying, that's always the key to success.

U

UNATTENDED Alzheimer's patients and those with dementia can get into dangerous situations. They should not be left unattended for one minute. Not only do they do funny things, like putting the newspaper in the freezer and taking off their clothes, but they also turn on the stove burners, leave the faucet running, drink toxic liquids, or wander off. I've cleaned up a lot of messes because I didn't jump up immediately and follow my husband when he headed for the kitchen. Jumping up saves you extra work. Close supervision can save your loved one's life, or your home.

UNAWARENESS of the gradual changes in a loved one can occur when you are closely involved. When our son lived in Atlanta, he came home to visit every few months. One time he said to me, "Mom, Dad's slipped a lot since the last time I was here." It brought me up short. I hadn't noticed a change, but Gary's remark made me stop and think. I realized he was right. I had blocked changes out on purpose because they were so hard to accept. Now,

Janice Hucknall Snyder

I am more observant and aware of little mental and physical changes.

It is important for you to be alert to changes, as you are the communicator between the patient and the doctor. You are the observer who is best able to inform the doctor on just what is going on with the patient. Some unfavorable changes are treatable through adjustments in medication. Your alertness could result in the patient's condition improving, making your burden easier.

UNDERSTANDING is the power to form reasoned judgments. Understanding is a powerful word when dealing with people from other countries in this world. It is a powerful word when dealing with individuals in our lives. Too often we are so sure of how we understand something that we can't open our minds long enough to hear what another person's understanding is. Are we afraid we might have to admit the other fellow has a point too? That is how conflicts are born in countries and in families. Dear Abby's column is full of the personal conflicts, misunderstandings and hurt feelings of people no longer speaking to one another. That is sad, but true.

You, as a caregiver, have a special need for understanding if your loved one has problems communicating. People who are unable to function normally aren't always responsive to the things that have to be done for and to them. They don't think people really understand just how terrible their world is, and they are probably right. Showing sympathy and having tolerance for your dependent's position helps to make for a closer relationship. When there is understanding, there is less stress, which is always beneficial to you both.

UNFAIRNESS is a bitter pill to swallow. Usually pretty early in our lives, we come to the realization that unfairness exists. If you think that your lot in life is unfair, think how your dependent must feel. Would you like to trade places? Life isn't always fair, there's no doubt about that. But when you let that negative thought distort your thinking, it can lead to negative actions.

Someone in our community just shot and killed a man walking along the beach with his fiancée for $20.00. That's what the man who was killed had in his wallet. I guess the killer thought life hadn't been fair to him. How tragic.

Whenever the word "unfair" starts intruding on my thinking, I immediately think of all the people I know whose lives have been dealt a lot more unfairness than mine.

UNNATURAL AND UNPLEASANT is how I would describe having to clean another person's private parts. This is something that never gets easier. It is vital that these areas are checked on a regular basis and kept clean. Urinary tract infections and rashes can be very painful to the patient, so extra care should be taken on your part to sanitize these areas thoroughly. Using rubber gloves helps a lot to get you through this process, especially when dealing with the dreaded diarrhea. Always coat red, irritated areas with a soothing petroleum jelly or cream.

UPSETS are upsetting. They will happen anyway. People usually cause them. That's upsetting too. Some people are experts at upsetting others; they know just the right words to set them off. Caregivers need to stay clear of those kinds of experts.

Have you ever noticed how the people who can upset you the most are those you love the most? It stands to reason. If a person didn't mean anything to you, nothing that person said could significantly hurt you. You and your dependent necessarily spend a great deal of time together, which can put undue strain on you both. When your dependent says things to upset you, it hurts. It makes tending to his/her needs more difficult for you. When you say things to upset your dependent, he/she feels helpless, guilty and sad.

When you truly love someone, you try extra hard and are extra careful not to say hurtful, upsetting things that will keep you from having that love returned. When there is togetherness, there are bound to be upsets. How you handle upsets is a real test of your maturity. The quicker you smooth things out, the quicker you both feel better.

URINE, urine everywhere, and boy, have I cleaned up my share. No matter how I try to catch it, in a plastic cut-off half gallon milk bottle (I've made several), in a store bought urinal, or in a Depends, surprises will happen.

Many years ago, when I was just a kid, knock knock jokes were all the rage. The only one I remember goes like this, "Knock knock."

"Who's there?"

"Peabody."

"Peabody who?

"Pea-bo-dy fence when nobody's looking." Yak, yak, yak! Boo hoo hoo. Because when I'm not looking, I usually wish I were. It isn't by the fence, but it could be on a rug, or in the bed (the Depends discarded on the floor), or in a waste paper basket. The latter is my preference, needless to say. In fact, finding it in the basket may even be my thrill for the day. Dealing with this unpleasantness is frustrating and exasperating, but I do survive it, barely. Keeping on my toes and knowing my husband's habits helps some, but in the middle of the night, all bets are off. I let tomorrow morning's surprises wait until tomorrow, because with a good night's sleep, I can handle anything. I keep a big box of Baking Soda handy for the rug, plastic bags in the waste basket, and moist disposable towelettes, talcum powder, ointment, towels, deodorants and a plastic hamper for wet sheets, all conveniently located. Most important, I keep my sense of humor ready at all times. Do you?

Janice Hucknall Snyder

V

VACATIONS away from the dependent are important for you for many reasons. The obvious ones being: a need for rest, a change in scenery, a chance to enjoy outside activities, and relief from stress and routine washing, cleaning and cooking. To me, none of the above reasons are as important as the one I'll mention next. Whether the vacation is three weeks or three hours, the time apart gives a brief sense of normalcy to your altered life style. It helps you to stay in touch with your own sense of identity. This is desperately needed, since your primary focus is on the constant needs of the ill person. Take advantage of every opportunity given to spend time away from home. It will help keep "burn out" away from your door.

VARIETY is the spice of life in more ways than the one generally meant by that statement. There needs to be a variety of activities for the ill person and for you to do. It is easy to get in a rut when living is restricted by handicaps. Stay clear of ruts; they are hard to get out of. Read different types of books, try new recipes for meals, get a new set of sheets for your bed, eat in a different room, start a new hobby; anything that stimulates the senses, takes the edge off a dull day, and helps to keep your spirits up.

VIDEOS, CDS AND DVDS are another wonderful way to get variety in your lives when going to the movies is out of the question. As I mentioned elsewhere, they are great for recording shows on TV that you miss when the dependent suddenly requires attention. Have you always dreamed of traveling the world? Rent tapes on all the different countries. They do a beautiful job of showing the highlights of each country and its people. They are for the armchair traveler, and you don't have to worry about drinking the water. There are wonderful travel videos for your viewing pleasure. No, it is not as exciting and wonderful as actually being there, but it is a whole lot cheaper and more convenient. Your luggage is safe and your feet appreciate you saving them wear and tear. Why not rent a different country every month? Having things like that to look forward to is a vital criterion for your mental survival.

VEGETABLES, some kids (and some adults) would say, are yucky. They are definitely not as yummy as lemon meringue pie, but they are an important part of one's diet. The rule of thumb with our kids was that they could each select one vegetable that they didn't have to ever eat. We thought that was fair, and it worked great. Many years later, they informed us that all of the vegetables they didn't like, they didn't eat. Some ended up in their napkins, or they would get a sudden urge to use the bathroom, in which case, the offending greens were actually flushed down the toilet. Our kids were good fakers; I never suspected.

A variety of vegetables are good for one's health, regularity, etc. Many years ago, President George Bush announced to the world that the one vegetable he avoided, at all costs, was broccoli. Well, it turns out that broccoli is a very important vegetable and should be eaten nearly every other day. It has been proven that it decreases the chance of colon cancer and other cancers. I'm sure that this is just another phase, since everything that is supposed to be good for us eventually is found to be bad for us, and vice versa. Just keep eating those greens until you hear differently. We don't want to overlook anything that's good for the patient and the caregiver.

VELCRO, oh, what a wonderful invention you are. This is especially so when the patient has Alzheimer's or some other form of dementia. Velcro is a real assist to the caregiver. It makes dressing and undressing the disabled a lot easier and quicker, especially if you have arthritis in your fingers. When my husband started having difficulty figuring out how to unbutton and unzip his pants, I installed Velcro tapes. This saved on "accidents" requiring the cleanup department, namely, me. Even if you have never sewed much, installing the tape is a fairly simple task. The backside on the Velcro tape is sticky, so it is easy to position the tape where the buttons were and then hem stitch around the edges of the tape. Anyone in a store where sewing materials are sold would be happy to show you how. The Velcro is more secure and the process is faster if a sewing machine is available to attach the tape, especially if revamping the patient's whole wardrobe.

VERTIGO is a very unpleasant sensation to experience and can be difficult to diagnose. In an older, ill person, it can be the cause of a bad fall, with the added complication of broken bones. Many different things can cause vertigo: fluid in the inner ear, a virus, certain drugs, double vision, brain tumors, clogged arteries, etc. A doctor, to determine just how serious the problem is, should always treat this condition early on. It is hard enough taking care of the patient without the added complication of broken bones to put further stress on you both.

VIAGRA is the wonder drug that puts a smile on lots of senior citizens' faces and the faces of many others who suffer from erectile dysfunction. See your doctor to get approval and be provided with a prescription for this uplifting drug.

VICTORY for the caregiver comes in the form of each day you survive without feeling defeated. Each day has its challenges, new and old problems, crises, demands and routines. When I "lay me down to sleep," I thank God I made it through another day victoriously. If it wasn't so victorious, I pray that tomorrow will be better. I go to sleep having faith that I'll survive no matter what tomorrow brings. That's a victory in itself.

VIGOROUS enthusiasm for living, no matter what the circumstances, can get you through a lot of bad stuff. It requires mental exercises for upbeat thoughts; it means being your own best pal. Patting yourself on the back when no one else is around to give a boost is okay too. Any action, within reason, that gives you a vigorous, upbeat attitude, does some good. We're talking survival here.

VIOLENCE is a word that connotes the things that nightmares are made of. One cannot pick up a newspaper or turn on a TV newscast without being confronted with it. We used to watch the news during dinner, but not anymore. Who needs graphic causes for indigestion?

On another level, some dependents with advanced Dementia can develop personality changes and psychotic behavior, which may even be violent in nature. I have mentioned elsewhere that when that happens, when you are unable to control the patient, it is necessary to put the person in a facility. There, he/she cannot be a danger to him/herself or others. It is a sad, but realistic, truth.

On still another level, if you are caring for your husband, that means he is unable to function as the "protector" in your home. Therefore, certain precautions should be maintained. We live in a lovely, small community, but drugs are everywhere now. Our township is not exempt from this cause for violence. Homes have been broken into and the owners robbed while they were asleep in their beds. Owning a gun has to be a personal decision. Short of that, I am careful to keep all doors locked and a large spray can by my bed. Supposedly, this spray would paralyze an intruder for twenty minutes, that is, if I aimed it in the right direction and wasn't too paralyzed with fear to push the button. Don't count on dialing 911 on your phone; intruders are very capable of cutting your phone lines. Many people use home alarm systems. They give some peace of mind, but are rough on a tight budget, which a lot of caregivers have. Constantly worrying about what could happen is a useless gesture loaded with stress. I've never given it space in my already overcrowded schedule of concerns, except when my next-door neighbor's house was robbed twice in two months. Gulp! Face the facts; don't be lax.

VIRUSES come around every year, especially in the winter. All dependents, older people and caregivers should get the vaccine. It is given in September and October and minimizes chances of getting a very serious illness that could result in a long recovery period or even death. Don't put it off.

VISE-LIKE GRIPS are hard to break out of. I used to hold my husband's hands when he walked because his feet freeze in place and he tends to lose his balance. Now, his fear of falling makes him extremely tense at times. When this first started occurring, his grip on my hands would become very strong and painful. I was barely able to free myself. To avoid this discomfort, I now grip his wrists to keep control. If you have a similar problem with your dependent, I think your fingers will appreciate avoiding the crunch. Grab those wrists.

VITAMINS should be taken daily for the three Vs, vim, vigor and vitality. The three Vs are all welcome energies that ward off fatigue and aid in the caregiver's survival. They are a definite asset in keeping you going when the going gets tough. How you feel and act affects everyone around you, most especially the person who is ill. The patient feels badly when he/she sees the person who is caring for him/her dragging from fatigue. So keep those vitamins going down.

VOICE inflection reflects inner calmness, tension, compassion, anger, tranquility, turmoil, joy and sadness. Babies learn to understand how parents are feeling by the tone in their voices long before they understand the language being spoken. Children sense it when parents are at odds. Though a word may never be spoken, they know before they are told that a divorce is pending.

One of my biggest failings as a caregiver is my inability to keep my emotions from showing in my voice. When I get impatient, excited or angry, my voice raises an octave and doubles in volume. To make matters worse, I have the kind of voice that you only want to have around when someone has driven off down the road and you need someone to holler, "Stop." Having admitted all that, I am not one who should be advising you to try to always speak in a calm, well-modulated tone of voice. But I do advise it, because loud vocalization can easily upset a person with dementia, and a disabled person is very sensitive to the meaning behind tone of voice. When there's a smile on your face, there will be a smile in your voice. This will keep your patient happy. When your patient is happy, you'll find the going easier. I don't mean to make it sound so simple, it isn't. It requires the patience of a saint, a heart of gold and the fortitude to persevere.

Janice Hucknall Snyder

WALKING is good exercise. If your patient is confined to a wheelchair, then do the walking for you both. Get outside in the fresh air and take deep breaths. Enjoy the change of view from four walls to scenes provided by Mother Nature. Weather permitting, make it a daily event.

Several years ago, we saw a man in our neighborhood walking briskly and taking long strides with his arms swinging in a wide arc. We had noticed because the man was so gaunt and pale he looked like he had one foot in the grave. We watched him go by every morning during the next year, and we observed an amazing transformation. He put on weight, developed leg and arm muscles, tanned and appeared ten years younger. He looked like a different man. So put on those walking shoes and get going.

WANDERING off can be a serious problem for the caregiver of an Alzheimer's or Dementia patient. It requires constant surveillance, which is tedious indeed. I've mentioned elsewhere the importance of the dependent wearing an identification bracelet. But this is small consolation if your loved one is missing. Put double locks on all doors leading outside, and keep them locked. Be sure all your neighbors have been made aware of your dependent's condition. The more people who are on the alert, the less chance there is of the patient getting very far from home. There's nothing more frightening than finding your dependent is not where you left him a few minutes before and, searching the house, coming up empty. That's rapid heartbeat time. I know. So keep eyes and ears open and stay close.

WEARINESS is no stranger to the caregiver. It's easy enough to say you shouldn't overdo it, but that's a joke. It is going to happen. On especially difficult days, weariness will set in. As I've mentioned elsewhere, learn to know when it's time to yell "Time." Call in family or friends to give you a break, even if only for a couple of hours. Take in a movie, relax in a hot tub or crash in your bed for a nap.

While I'm working, my husband stays in a day care center. I pick him up at 6 p.m. Just recently they have started a new feature, sponsored by a Christian group of people. Now, the last Friday in each month is "Caregiver's night out." There is no additional charge. A light supper is served the clients, and we pick up our loved ones at 9:30 p.m.. My first thought was that it would be too long of a day for my husband. They reminded me that he sleeps a lot and isn't aware of time, adding that I needed a break. I had to agree with that. My first "night out," I stayed in town, got to swim laps, and met my cousin, Caroline, for a movie and dinner. It was a real treat. Our next special Friday is one week away, and I can hardly wait. It is nice to have something to look forward to like that. What a wonderful, thoughtful gift some caring people have given to us. I hope that wherever you are living, someone or some group has arranged something similar for you. If not, get the ball rolling yourself. Be in touch with all the churches in your area. This could be a meaningful joint effort for the good of all.

WEATHER is a mood changer. Dreary, overcast rainy days can be depressing, especially several in a row. Hot, humid days are enervating and can make one short-tempered. Plan special indoor activities that are fun to do and lift one's spirits on those days. Computer and video games are not only exciting, but also good for improving coordination. Save a special book you want to read for these occasions too, or a jigsaw puzzle. Writing about your thoughts and feelings is always beneficial. The main thing is to keep busy with uplifting activities so that the ole miserable weather syndrome doesn't hang around too long.

WELL-BEING, in Webster's, is described as "the state of being healthy, happy and free from want." Wow, that is a tall order for most of us, but it's certainly something to strive for in our lives.

As a caregiver, you know all too well the importance of staying healthy. Be thankful for every day that you are.

Happiness is a state of mind that is only achieved through your own personal acceptance of what your life is all about.

Free from want? How many people can honestly say they are? Even the very rich don't always get what they really want. I guess the only way one can be free from want is to be content with simple wants.

The state of your well-being is important, because it directly affects your ability to deal with whatever you have to deal with.

WHEELCHAIRS give the disabled a means of getting around when mobility becomes limited. There are many different types to choose from, depending on the mobility of the patient. A lighter weight folding chair is easier for a woman or older man to lift into a car.

WHINING patients try one's patience. Many older people develop a whiny way of speaking to solicit attention and sympathy. It seems to me that women are more inclined to do this than men. If your dependent is a whiner, you need to nip it in the bud. Tell the whiner that you will answer their question or get the item they want when the words are repeated in a normal tone of voice. The sentence may be repeated three or four more whining times before your dependent realizes that you are not going to respond until his/her voice has a pleasant tone. This method does work, but consistency is important to keep the whiner from reverting back to this unpleasant habit.

WHY? That is the question. How often during a lifetime do we ask ourselves why, or why me? Why anybody? Sometimes, even years later, I've gotten the answer. I have found understanding and even some good that came out of a not so good experience.

Caregivers, and their dependents especially, have good reason to wonder why. But there is nothing gained from that question. In fact, it can lead to depression sprinkled with self-pity. It is best to accept what cannot be changed and to try to keep an ongoing optimistic attitude. Ours not to wonder why, but to try, try, try.

WILLPOWER is what it takes to be in control of our actions and emotions. When I think of willpower, I automatically think of dieting. That is the area where the strength of one's willpower separates the fat from the thin. It takes a lot of will power to control your temper, stay on a budget, and stop over-eating, drinking or smoking. It takes a lot of willpower to not spread a rumor and to keep smiling when the bottom falls out. Where does willpower come from? I think it comes from a strong determination and conviction deep within your spirit about what is right and wrong. Sheer willpower gives you the strength to overcome, to survive.

WITHDRAWAL happens in cases of depression. People with physical or mental problems are prone to depression, and therefore to withdrawal. When the need for sleep increases several hours, it should be considered a sign of withdrawal. There are some situations you need help with, and this is one of them. A doctor should be consulted at once. This condition requires professional treatment. Sharing the responsibility in dealing with this condition eases your burden.

WONDERING what will happen to you and your dependent in the future? That can be agonizing. When the foreseeable future doesn't look bright, negative thoughts tend to seep in. Avoid such thoughts. After all, nobody really knows what the future holds. New scientific discoveries are being made all the time. Perhaps the next one will help your loved one. Hold that thought. Just wonder about what is happening to you today, this minute. That's all any of us have anyway.

WORDS are the way most people communicate. The effect of words spoken by one individual to another can be uplifting or devastating.

When I was a kid, a favorite response to unkind words was always, "sticks and stones can break my bones, but words can never hurt me." I never gave that saying much thought when I yelled it back to someone. Then one day I realized how wrong that saying was. Words did hurt when unkind remarks or slurs were made to me or someone I loved. They hurt deep inside me. Children say a lot of cruel things, so do adults. It's a real downer. Try to keep encouraging, nice words coming forth for the benefit of your dependent and for your own self-worth.

WORKING is a necessary part of surviving. It can be difficult at best, but when you are a caregiver, it requires great fortitude and management of time. I drop my husband off at the day care facility every morning at 8 a.m. and pick him up by 6 p.m. Actually, working is a great help to my survival. I love my job, which is a big plus. It also enables me to communicate with many people and it gives me needed time for tending to business affairs and shopping. All the remainder of my time is spent with my husband. He requires my constant attention and cannot be left alone. On the minus side of working, it is difficult to rise and shine some mornings when I've been up two or three times with my husband during the night. Still, I recommend that you have some form of outside activity, maybe even a part-time job. I feel it gives balance and diversity to an otherwise confined and totally restricted life. It keeps you from becoming totally wiped out, which is what twenty-four hours a day of care for your dependent can do to you.

WORLD HAPPENINGS are mostly bad news: plane crashes, wars, starving children, murders, etc. Caregivers have a great, tragic burden to bear of their own, so a daily dose of the "world" is, at times, more than you need to deal with. A good alternative is to turn off the TV news and turn on a favorite radio station that plays soothing music. We were in the habit of listening to the news at dinnertime, but not anymore. Music is better for the digestion.

In the "olden" days, people had no way of hearing about catastrophes in the next state, much less around the world.

I really think they were better off. Now, it's instant tragedies with graphic details. We do need to care about other people and the problems of the world, but it can be overwhelming at times when you are dealing with personal sadness daily. So, survival requires you to know when the saturation point has been reached in viewing gross world conditions. Pushing the off button on the remote control takes care of the problem with the greatest of ease. Do it; it's an uplifting experience.

WORRYING can make you sick. How do you deal with it? I just read an item in the paper, and I quote, "A study found that people who took time to write down their worries on paper not only felt better about themselves, but actually strengthened their body's immune systems." How about that? The theory is that by expressing oneself, even if only in writing, one can relieve stress. I'm a living testimonial to that. Writing this book has been a great outlet for my feelings and has helped me, in many ways, to endure.

As for worrying, fortunately for me, as I stated earlier, when I was twenty-two years old I almost died from a pregnancy. I say fortunately because it changed my whole outlook on life. It gave me a real awareness of just how precious life is. Since then, my philosophy has been to live each day as though it could be my last. I have gotten a lot of mileage out of life using that principle. That experience, so long ago, gave me a whole new appreciation for the value of time. It also changed my thinking on what is truly important in life. I had been a "worry-wart" until my close call. After that, things that had seemed so important, no longer were. Then and there I decided to worry a whole lot less about material things. Worrying doesn't really help anything, but can make you physically ill; then you really have something to worry about.

Janice Hucknall Snyder

When you have a loved one who is seriously ill, you do worry about him or her, of course. Health problems are the exception to the "no worry" philosophy. But I don't let myself worry constantly; it would be unhealthy. What I cannot change, I turn over to God. He can handle it much better than I.

WORTH is the value placed on someone, or something. Some people value things more than people, robbing and killing anyone to get the things they want. Life has no value to them.

Actually, the worth of a human being is beyond any given value; it is priceless. All human beings should cherish each other. Needless to say, that is a Utopian point of view. Wouldn't the world be a wonderful place if it were so?

As a caregiver, you know the value of life; you spend a great deal of your time caring for and preserving someone else's. But in so doing, you can neglect taking care of yourself. Breaks in the schedule, a night out, pacing yourself, getting enough shut-eye and being alert to signs of fatigue, are just a few of the things you can do to show you value your own self-worth.

WRITING is a way of expressing yourself. It gets inner feelings out in the open, where they can be looked at more objectively. Caregivers need to recognize and deal with their emotions on a regular basis to keep steam from building up. Write down those thoughts; it is emotionally healthy. You can always burn up your journal, but you can't take back unkind words that burst forth when frustration reaches a boiling point. So grab a pen and get busy.

X

X marks the spot where you are right now in dealing with surviving as a caregiver. How do you think you are holding up? On a scale of one to ten, how would you say you are handling everything? Give yourself a six or better? Good for you. If you think you rate a four or less, you are sinking fast. It's time to get help from someone or somewhere. Don't dilly-dally. Survival is the name of the game. It's a good idea to stop once in a while and take stock of just how you feel mentally and physically. It helps to put things in perspective.

X-RAYS are necessary in diagnosing many conditions: fractures, breast lumps, lung disease, brain tumors, etc. Yes, sometimes X-Rays are prescribed to protect the doctor from the risk of a malpractice suit. And yes, that is part of the reason health insurance is so high.

Sometimes it is good to confront your doctor with the issue of whether or not an X-ray is really necessary. My husband had a CAT scan when he was diagnosed with Parkinson's Disease; it was negative. Then, five years later, he had another scan when there were signs of Dementia;

it was negative. The following year, a Neuro-Psychologist evaluated him, and Parkinson's Dementia was confirmed. That doctor ordered still another CAT scan. I questioned my husband's Neurologist. I asked him what difference another scan at this point would make. They had already ruled out a brain tumor, and another CAT scan would change nothing. He agreed completely and cancelled the test.

Don't be afraid to question why procedures are being done. It is your right and, in fact, your responsibility. When I was in the hospital following the birth of my first child, a nurse brought me pills every night. I asked what they were for. The nurse gave a vague answer like, "Oh, to make you feel better." I inquired further. It turned out that pill was to dry up my milk. I said to the nurse, "Well, that is just great, since I plan to nurse my baby."

No one had even bothered to ask me my wishes concerning this matter. Nursing your baby was not as popular at that time, so it was assumed I wouldn't nurse. Lucky for me, I asked in time. My daughter was happy about that too.

Never hesitate to ask questions about procedures and medications. Doctors and nurses are human, and, therefore, not perfect. They get exhausted, have personal problems, and have days when they don't feel in top form. They have days when they are capable of making questionable decisions. Your questions act as a safeguard in confirming and verifying the instructions given. It can make a difference in the quality of care your loved one gets. If your doctor gets impatient and offended by your questions, find another doctor. You have enough pressure on you without having to deal with a physician who doesn't give satisfactory answers and have the patient's welfare at heart.

X-Y-Z is a nice method I have of alerting a patient to the fact that his zipper is open. I say, "Do you know what X-Y-Z means?"

When they reply, "No," I explain that it means, "Examine Your Zipper," which they hurry to do. If the person already knows what X-Y-Z means, the response is a quick zip to correct the problem. It is a smooth way to handle this delicate matter and usually gets a laugh. I know this has nothing to do with your survival, but since the Xs are so brief, I thought I'd add this tidbit of trivia.

Janice Hucknall Snyder

Y

YEARNINGS are natural feelings in all people. As a caregiver, your life has to be so focused, so confined with another person that you are bound to have strong yearnings. Don't dismiss these desires as something that can never come to pass. Always keep your dreams and hopes alive with a positive attitude. When an opportunity presents itself to do something you've always yearned to do, go for it. Where there's a will, there's a way.

YELLING is good for the lungs and for releasing tension. It isn't good when it is directed at the ill person, though. Unfortunately, it's usually something that the ill person does that makes you want to yell the most.

Sometimes, in a moment of desperation, I find myself yelling something like, "Why did you do that?"

In the case of my husband, it's a stupid question. He really doesn't know why he does a lot of the things he does. I do feel badly when I yell, and naturally, it upsets him. But still, sometimes I just have to get the frustration out then and there. The need is pretty great when I can't wait until I'm in the shower. Don't be too hard on yourself if you find yourself yelling at times; let 'er rip. Sometimes, your needs really do outweigh the needs of the dependent. Those needs must be met in order to survive. If your yelling becomes an hourly need, then it's time to yell for help.

YELLOW BRICK ROADS lead to the Land of Oz, where all of our wishes are granted. It's another wonderful fairy tale. Everyone lives happily ever after. But in the real world, the way gets bumpy, the gold gets tarnished and the yellow brick road can lead to a dead end.

Caregivers and their dependents have special wishes too. How nice it would be if you could just visit the great Oz and, with a loud bang, clang or click of the heels, have your wishes come true. But, just as in the Wizard of Oz, if you look within yourself, you may find the answer is already there, just waiting to be recognized. A peaceful spirit within brings true happiness.

YESTERDAY all my sorrows seemed so far away, so sang The Beatles. Yesterdays are the memories of today. The sorrows of today, they too will pass away into yesterdays. Happy, glorious memories are a wonderful thing to stir up when the present is a sad time. But don't stir up the sad parts, let them pass away. Don't recall regrets that will haunt you. Do recall the miracles of life that have blessed you and yours. Keep yesterdays in the proper perspective, living each day as it is given and being thankful.

YOGA is a system of discipline and meditation. I found this explanation in the dictionary, as I am not a student of Yoga. However, my sister has practiced it for many years and found it very meaningful and fulfilling. I'm sure if we didn't live 1,000 miles apart, I would have had her teach me how to practice some of those disciplines and meditations.

Meditation would be very helpful in controlling stress and emotions in your life. Find time each day to be alone in a quiet place. Empty your mind of all thoughts, and then visualize a place of serene beauty for 15 minutes. This practice would be very beneficial to any person living in today's fast-paced environment.

"**YOU**" is a poem by an unknown author that was given to me by my dear Aunt Zaza when I was twelve years old. It is in a lovely frame, and I have cherished it for many years. It always made me feel better to read it. I would like to share it with you.

You

Sometimes when the shadows cross my path,
As shadows sometimes do,
I reach my hand across the mist
And touch the hand of you.

I know the sun is in the sky.
I know true love is true.
But how it comforts in the dark
To touch the hand of you.

It helps to have a special thought or saying that gives you reassurance when you are upset, hurt or afraid.

Janice Hucknall Snyder

Z

ZEAL is persistence, a fervent devotion to a cause. The caregiver's cause is keeping their loved one comfortable, clean and cheerful. To do this with zeal requires deep devotion. It is a challenge. It takes true grit, but the rewards are great. The satisfaction of knowing you have helped to ease another person's burden is what gives meaning and worth to your own existence.

ZENITH is reaching the highest point, right up there at the top. A lot of times, as a caregiver, you feel like you've reached the bottom. That's more familiar territory. But remember, when you reach the bottom, there is only one way to go, and that is up. The more positive you are in your thoughts and actions, the more variety you develop in your daily life. That gives you the boost you need to be right up there, reaching for the stars again.

ZERO is nothing, but being a caregiver is something. There is nothing about this labor of love that is easy. It is a calling you can be proud of. It stretches you to the limit in many directions: physically, spiritually, mentally and emotionally. On a scale from zero to ten, I would give all caregivers a big ten.

ZEST does for living what spices do for food. Jazz it up. Make it full of flavor. Without zest in our lives, we merely exist.

You don't have time for zest in your life, you say? Conditions are too sad and dreary to be enthusiastic about anything, you say? You are too tired all the time to feel zesty, you say?

I hope you don't say those things after reading this book, because keeping your spirits up is what this book is all about. Laughter is the best medicine of all for whatever ails everyone. So bring on the clowns. Free yourself up. Put some zest in your life. It will make your loved one feel better too, because a happy spirit is contagious.

ZIPPERS are a closing, one that you check on frequently if your dependent is a forgetful person. You can also replace zippers with Velcro to make opening and closing items easier on yourself.

~~~~~~~~~~~~~~~~~~~~~~~

In Closing

With that, I shall conclude my alphabetical list of words for the caregiver's survival. I hope your journey with me has given you a healthy attitude, hope, help, understanding and peace of mind. God Bless.

Janice Hucknall Snyder

POSTSCRIPT

Richard and I were 48 at the onset of his illnesses, depression, mental breakdown, Parkinson's disease and dementia. He was my inspiration during the 20 years I was his caregiver. The hardest period for me, as caregiver, were the last two months of his life because he had to spend them in a nursing home. Richard passed away peacefully at the age of 68. However, I had already done all of my grieving long before then. I rejoiced that Richard's sweet spirit was finally free. I still swim laps for 50 minutes, three times a week. I miss my dear, sweet husband seven days a week.

Janice Hucknall Snyder

Select MSI Books

Self-Help Books

A Woman's Guide to Self-Nurturing (Romer)

Creative Aging: A Baby Boomer's Guide to Successful Living (Vassiliadis & Romer)

Divorced! Survival Techniques for Singles over Forty (Romer)

How to Be a Good Mommy When You're Sick: A Guide to Motherhood with Chronic Illness (Graves)

Lessons of Labor: One Woman's Self-Discovery through Labor and Motherhood (Aziz)

Living Well with Chronic Illness (Charnas)

Publishing for Smarties: Finding a Publisher (Ham)

The Marriage Whisperer: How to Improve Your Relationship Overnight (Pickett)

The Rose and the Sword: How to Balance Your Feminine and Masculine Energies (Bach & Hucknall)

The Widower's Guide to a New Life (Romer)

Widow: A Survival Guide for the First Year (Romer)

Inspirational and Religious Books

A Believer-Waiting's First Encounters with God (Mahlou)

A Guide to Bliss: Transforming Your Life through Mind Expansion (Tubali)

El Poder de lo Transpersonal (Ustman)

Everybody's Little Book of Everyday Prayers (MacGregor)

Joshuanism (Tosto)

Puertas a la Eternidad (Ustman)

The Gospel of Damacus (O. Imady)

The Seven Wisdoms of Life: A Journey into the Chakras (Tubali)

When You're Shoved from the Right, Look to Your Left: Metaphors of Islamic Humanism (O. Imady)

Memoirs

Blest Atheist (Mahlou)

Forget the Goal, the Journey Counts . . . 71 Jobs Later (Stites)

Healing from Incest: Intimate Conversations with My Therapist (Henderson & Emerton)

It Only Hurts When I Can't Run: One Girl's Story (Parker)

Las Historias de Mi Vida (Ustman)

Losing My Voice and Finding Another (C. Thompson)

Of God, Rattlesnakes, and Okra (Easterling)

Road to Damascus (E. Imady)

Foreign Culture

Syrian Folktales (M. Imady)

The Rise and Fall of Muslim Civil Society (O. Imady)

Thoughts without a Title (Henderson)

Psychology/Philosophy

Road Map to Power (Husain & Husain)

Understanding the People around You: An Introduction to Socionics (Filatova)

Humor

Mommy Poisoned Our House Guest (C. B. Leaver)

The Musings of a Carolina Yankee (Amidon)

Other

365 Teacher Secrets for Parents: Fun Ways to Help Your Child in Elementary School (McKinley & Trombly)

The Subversive Utopia: Louis Kahn and the Question of National Jewish Style in Jerusalem (Sakr)